This is It

Enlightenment with CYoga

This is It

Enlightenment with CYoga

Catherine Foroughi

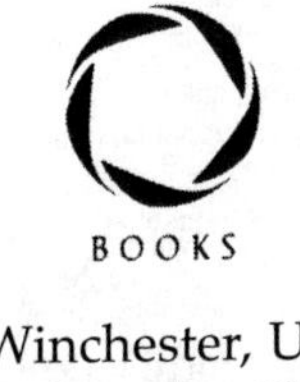

Winchester, UK
Washington, USA

First published by O-Books, 2012
O-Books is an imprint of John Hunt Publishing Ltd., Laurel House, Station Approach,
Alresford, Hants, SO24 9JH, UK
office1@o-books.net
www.o-books.com

For distributor details and how to order please visit the 'Ordering' section on our website.

ISBN: 978 1 84694 833 6

A CIP catalogue record for this book is available from the British Library.

Design: Lee Nash

Printed in the USA by Edwards Brothers Malloy

This is It

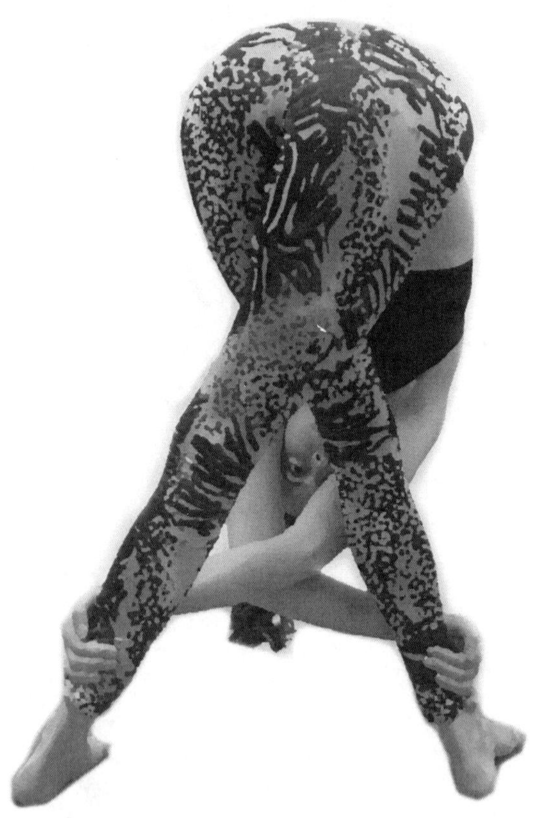

Welcome

This is I.
This is It II (aye aye) Enlightenment With CYoga!
This is a Gift for understanding yoga and Enlightenment, even if not interested in "asanas" on the mat.
This is sage wisdom presented in an indescribable prophetic and beautiful style.

This is the Guide for anyone *that* allows natural understanding from the teacher within and a relaxation in *That* space to manifest unashamedly.
This is Yoga!

I play with words and see and work with words such as *This* and *That that* share an eternal meaning.
See if *This* and *That's* meaning arises naturally.

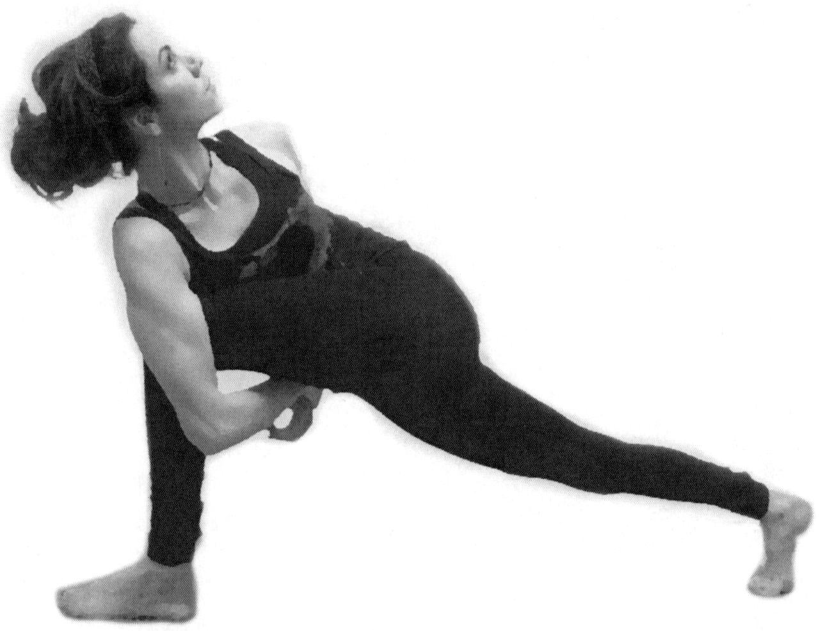

Ode on Improvement

There is no improvement in *This* moment
There is no improvement on *This* moment
See through any sense of "oh yeah, Now I'm more agile, a better player, more flexible, cleverer etc. etc."
What is the comparison with?

Can one see *that* with a sense of comparison it could always appear *that* one is improving
Keep it fresh.
If fresh there is no comparison - there is only now
Is *this* clear?

Understand *this*.
I understand! Everyone understands?!

There is an optical illusion with two shapes. The one in front always appears bigger than the one behind.
With measurements they are the same size and in the same place.
One is not behind or in front of the other.

If you (or is it I?!1) mention improvement do I teach yoga? How ridiculous is *That*? Will you ever learn? When? *This* is it.

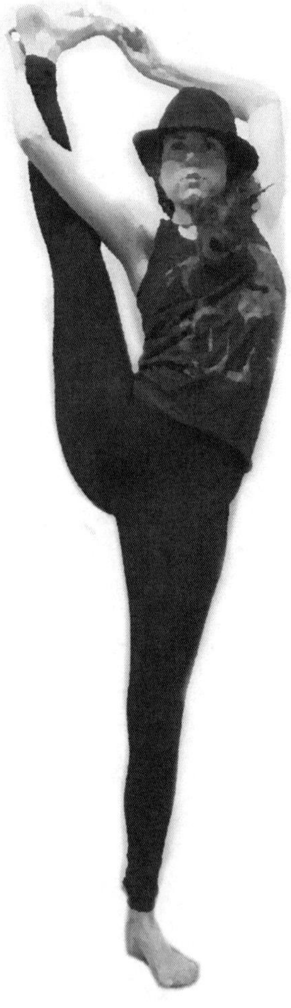

This is important or maybe not at all.

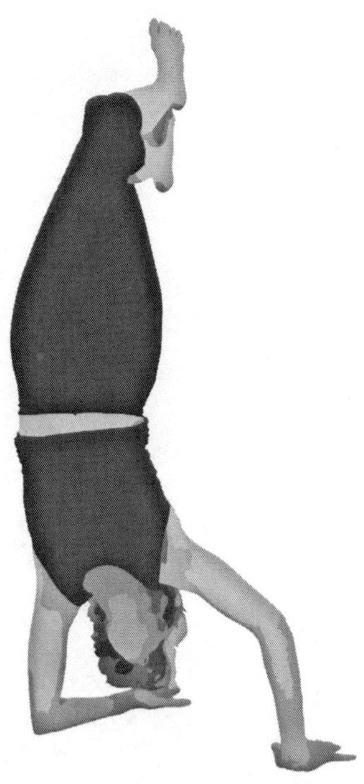

By(e) the way do you have *This* Is It: Enlightenment With CYoga.

Multiple meanings - I love them. *That* is me!

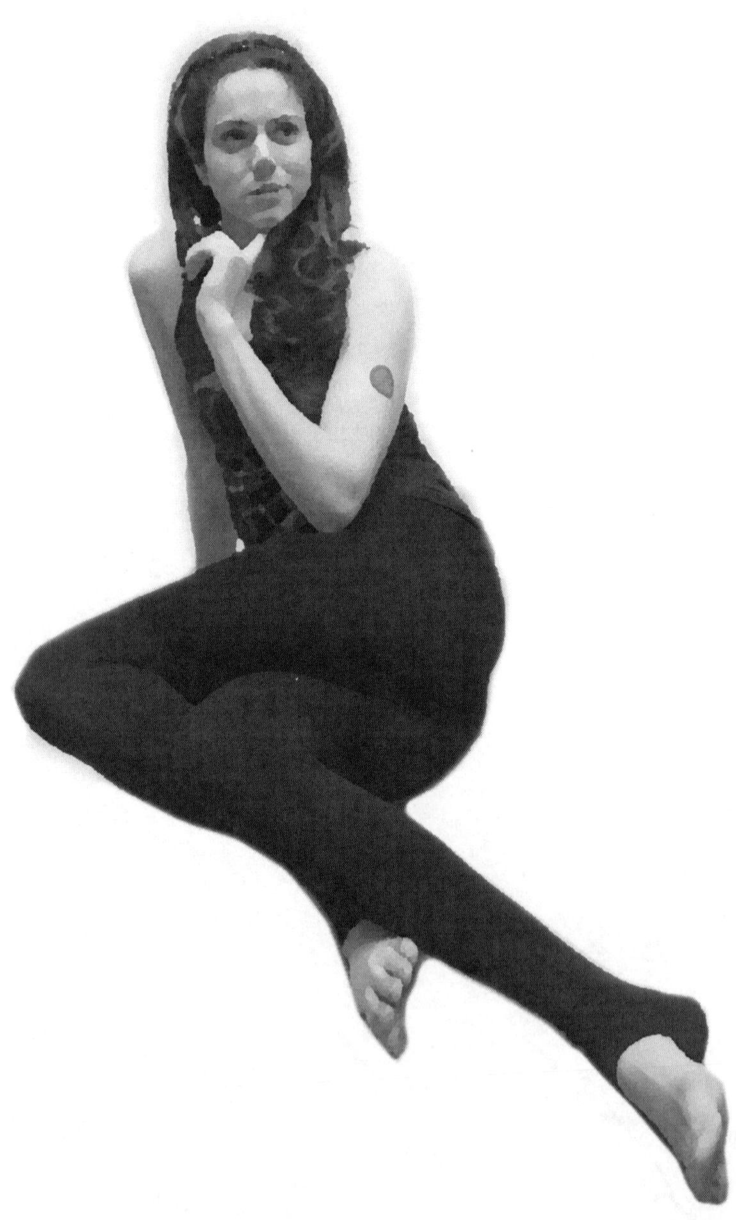

Ok come and see me for a yoga lesson! When shall we arrange it?!

Should I teach or show *this* understanding and/or allow it to emerge from within?!
Everything now is as it is!
If one gets *that* one is fundamentally free.
Comparison is not It.
Feel free and play with it all. (when?)
This is not for something else.
One is always free now.

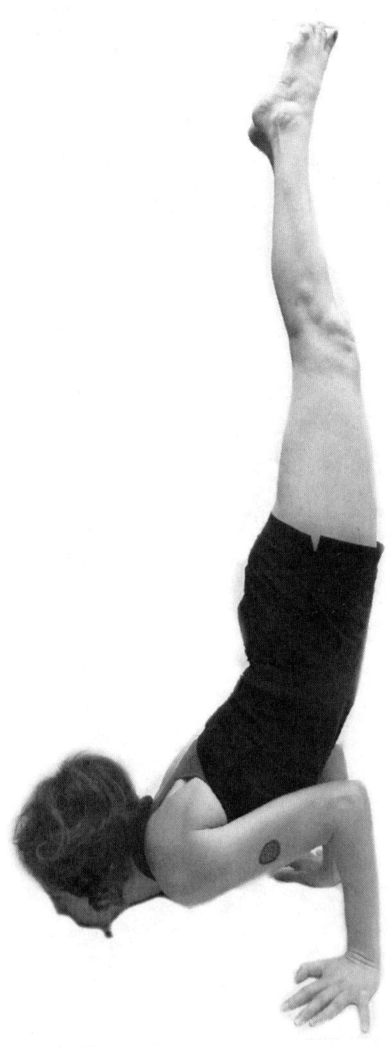

Free of any sense of improvement.
Yeah I'm improving or oh I used to be able to do *this* before can present.
Does one believe one improves?
Does one believe one gets worse?!
Does one pick n' choose what feelings one believes?

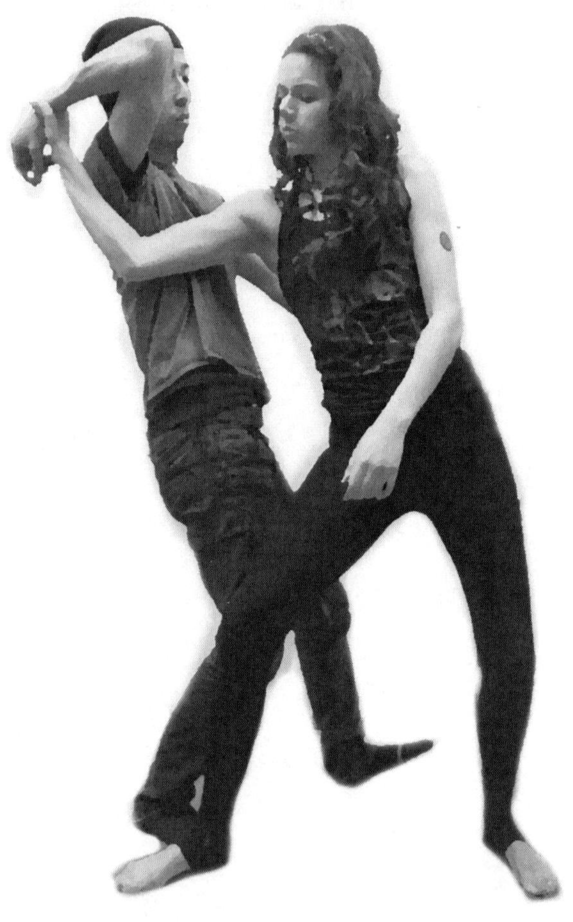

I = always No.1.
I am the winner!
That cannot be improved on.
Who wants t(w)o be No.2?

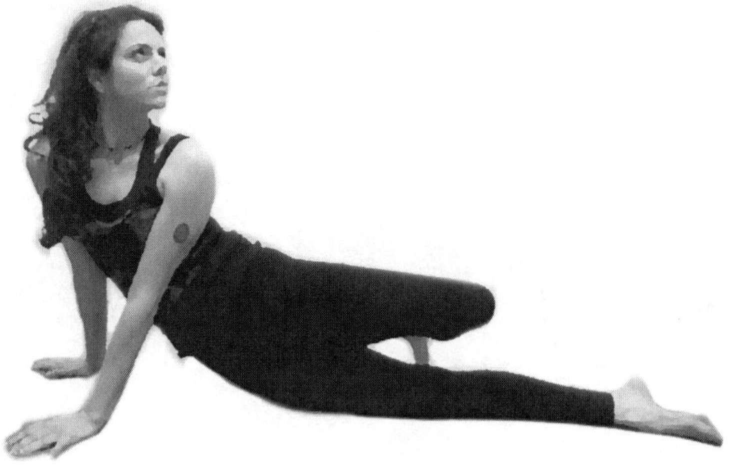

Q - Ok- what's the game?!

A- *This* is the *This* is It Game.

In answer to (nearly) all questions the answer is *This* is It.

Q -What are the *This* is It questions?

A - *This* is It!

Q - ok, ok. By the way are you going to the party….what did you do *this* weekend….what do you want for dinner…..?

A - *This* is It?!

Be. *This* is It is much simpler than explaining why brussell sprouts are what I like/ dislike; don't fancy getting on a train to Scotland where the party is supposedly; or discovering why the Buddhist needs practise appearing more confused than enlightened or why I like fluorescent pink.

The *This* is It Game is simple. One knows *This* is the only moment and It is as it is.

Q - When do we play *this* game?

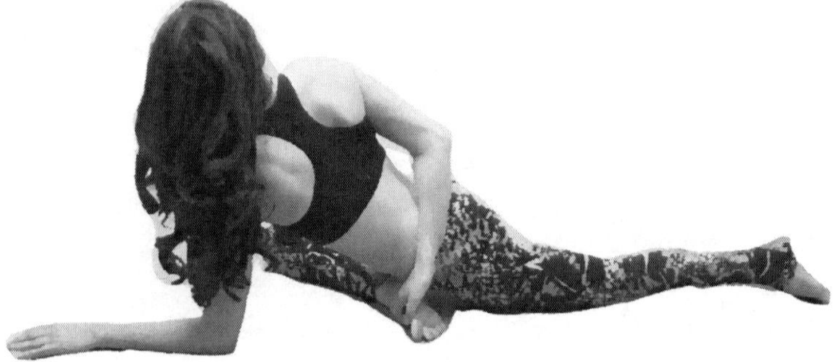

Yeah, there is a difference between just *This*

And "getting out of the ".
Did I introduce a ?

Nah.

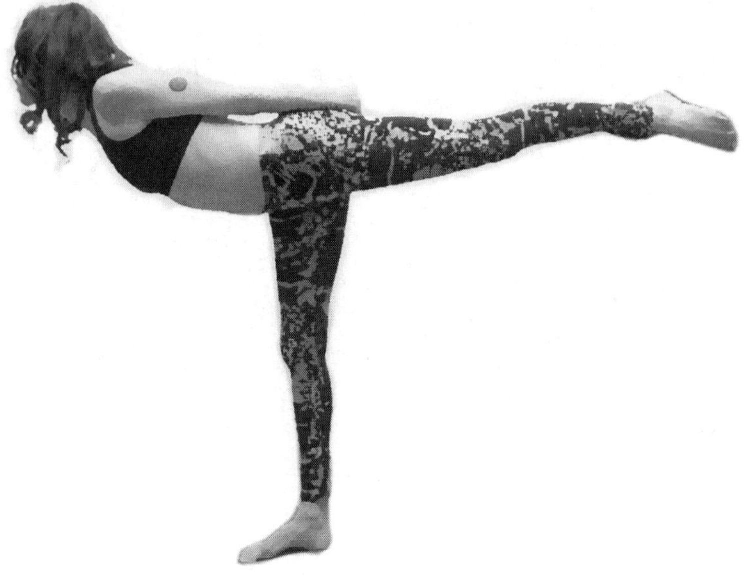

I am yoga.

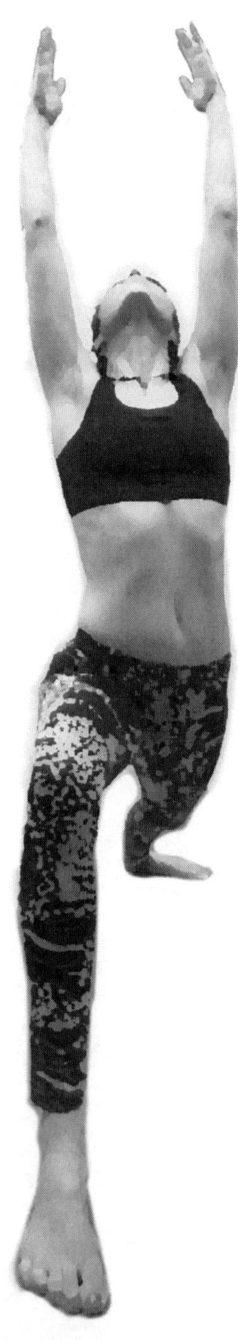

One experience's yoga from One sense. I.

It is funny seeing quotes with names and references such as ancient 19th century master. Are they genius? I wrote them!

"Now there is no subject and object". 21st century yoga genius

What is the experience now?
Is *this* it or is there a feeling *that* oh yes *that* experience sounds right?

One creates all Now.

I am Ramana, John, Tony (am I still PM?)(footnote 1), Kate and Katie.

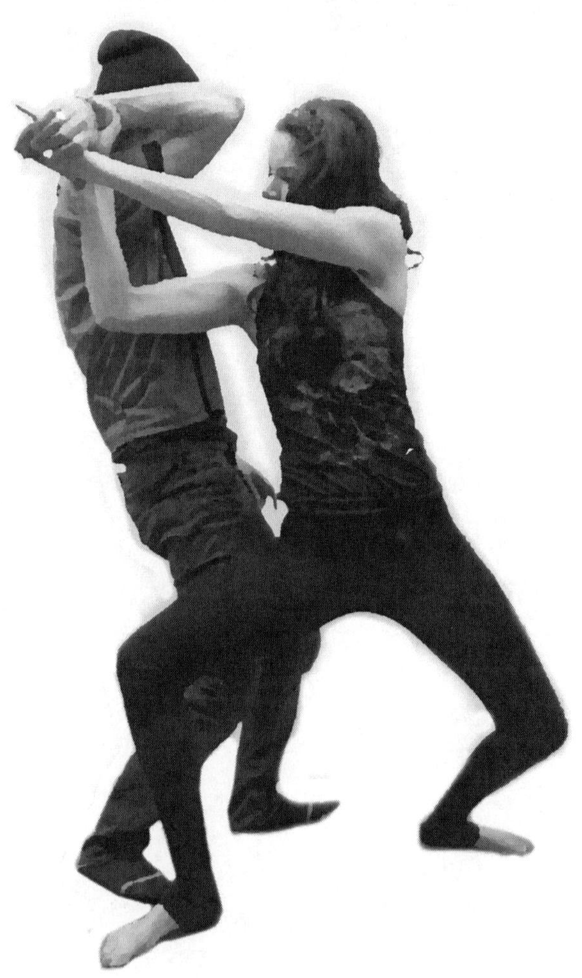

Do you agree with my words?!
By the way any sense of disagreement is a duality.
Oh well. Bring on the duel.
Shall we make it three just for fun?
Or perhaps fore?
It is as it is.
Whatever.

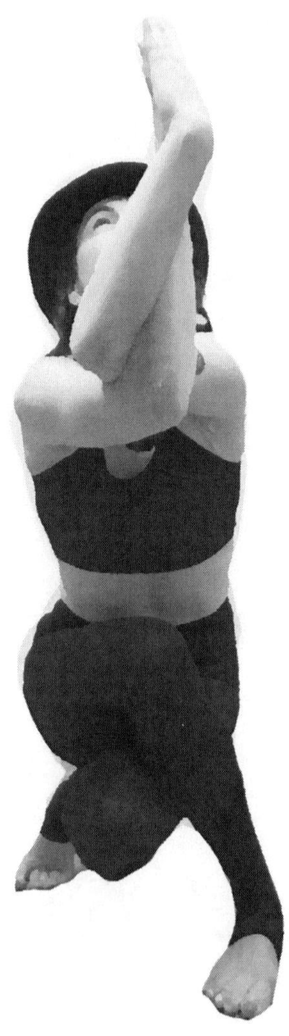

There is no joke.
Who's telling the joke?
Who's the recipient of the joke?
What's the subject of the joke?
Am I laughing?

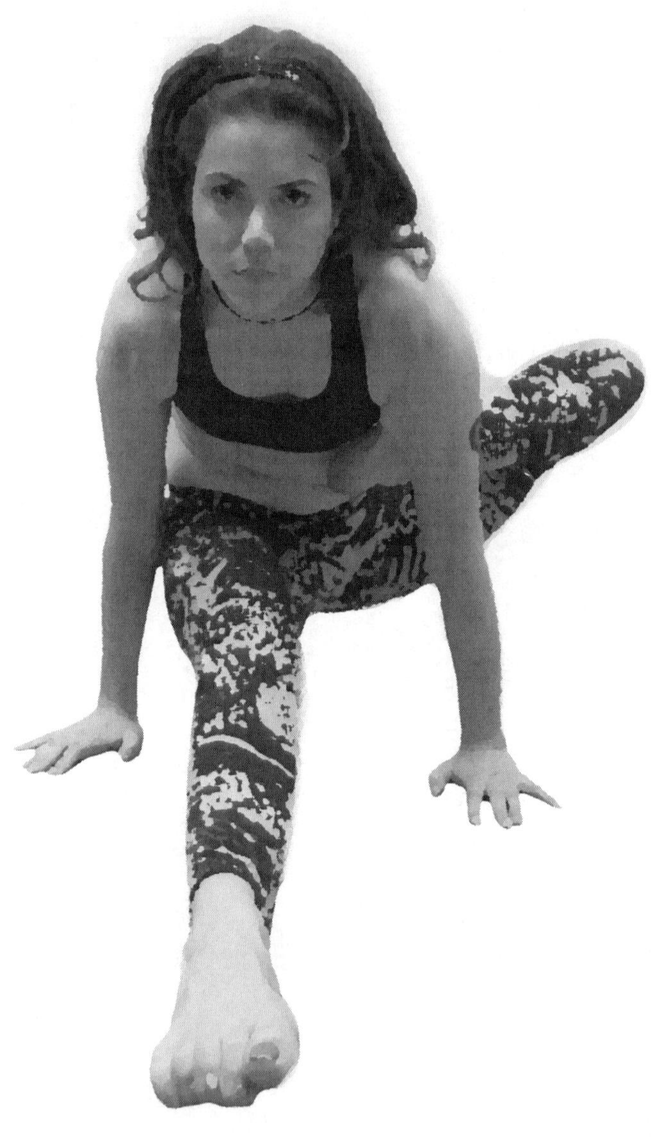

Why the question mark (?)!
See 1.
I am my editor,
I am you.
You are the editor.
You are I.

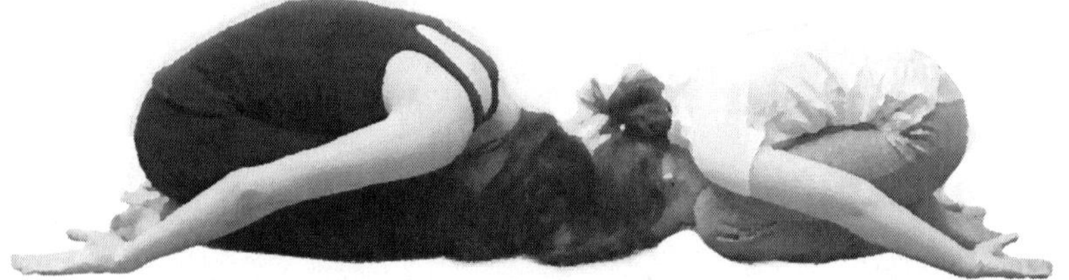

Ban "how are you?".
I am here.
I am present.
Do I really care how you are?
Who are you?
Do you look I(ll)?!
I can see you are present.
My eye is everywhere.

See the humour of/in word arrangements such as; when do I see you next; when do we next meet up; see you Monday or it will be sunny tomorrow ....; and THE WORST how long have you been practicing (uggggggggggh) yoga.

I am with you Now.
Is now Monday?
The weather I is as it is.
I do not practice yoga.

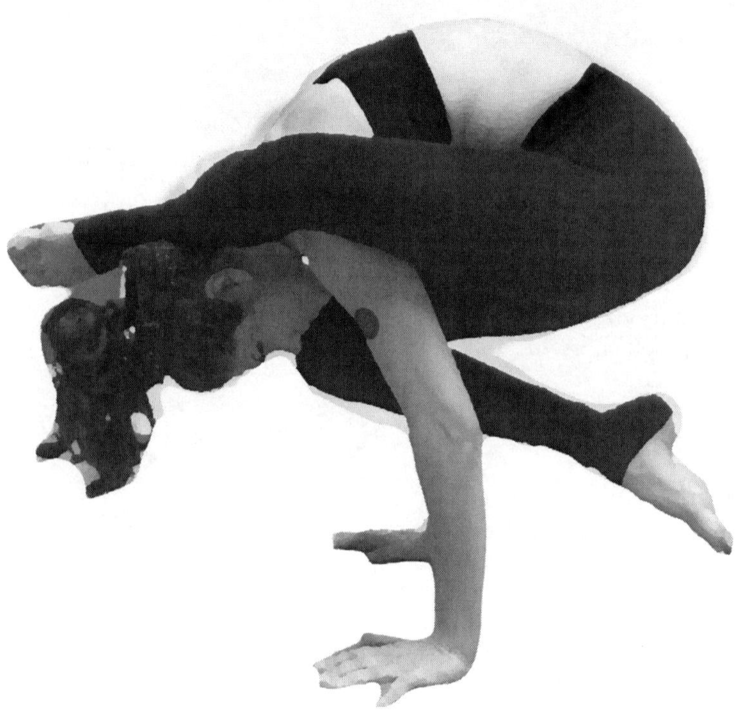

It is not practice *that* makes me lithe (legs behind head at *this* moment), gorgeous, talented, enlightened, grace, elegant, perfect/ present.

This is me naturally.

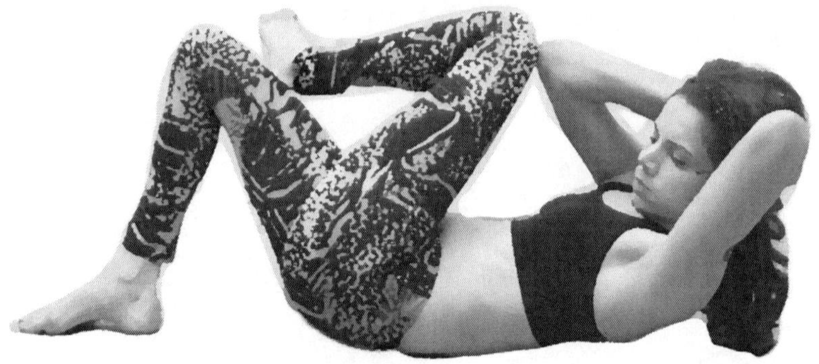

What is real knowledge?
What is truth?
Does one believe *that* seeing without thoughts and feelings one sees clearly?
What Is seen?
Does one see something real?
Is there only I?!
Remember maya?
Who is Maya?!

(She is Ralph's sister - ok I joke.)

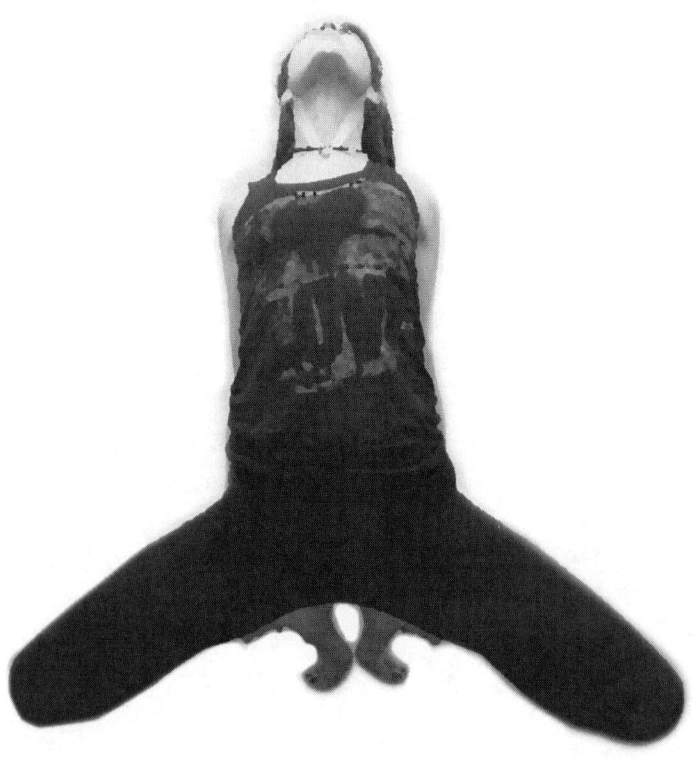

Nirvana is Here Now
This is not positive karma.
Is reading *this* nirvana?!1
If not now when?

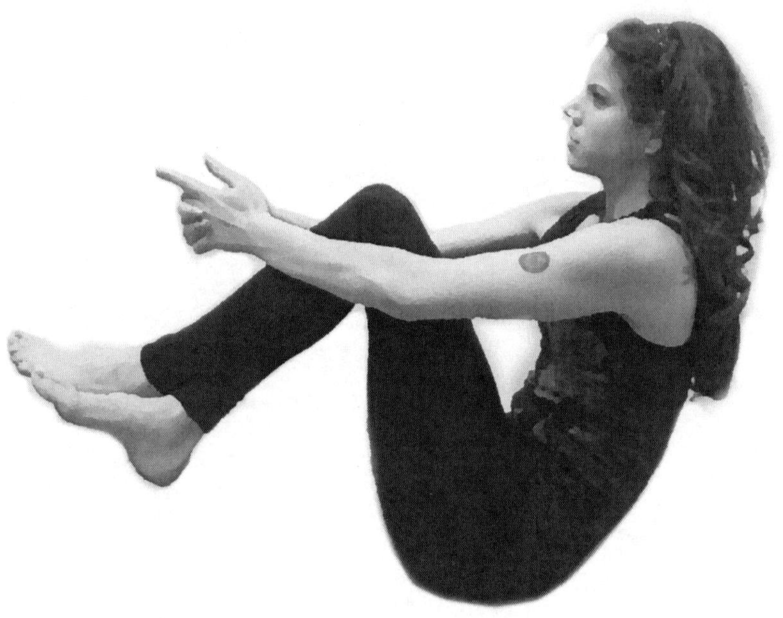

You know everything

i) One can only learn what one always knows.
If it is known now it is always known.
See?
This is a pointer *that* it is only for now.
This is a pointer *that* there is only now.

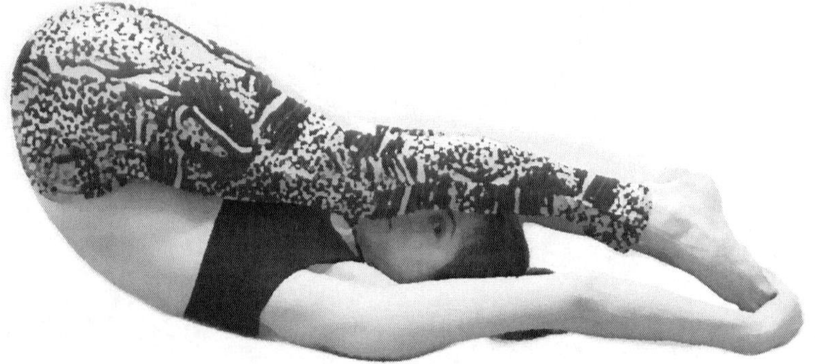

Is *this* book enlightenment?!
It is all yoga.
Does om shanti shanti shanti sound enlightening?
Does it?!
Is it just maya?
Actually it is.
God bless Dharma.
There are no sacred cows.
I can play with *this* and *that*.
This is It.
Thank God for oneness.
Who is God?
Me?!
And you! Yippee.
Thank God for oneness.
Is there a point? See.

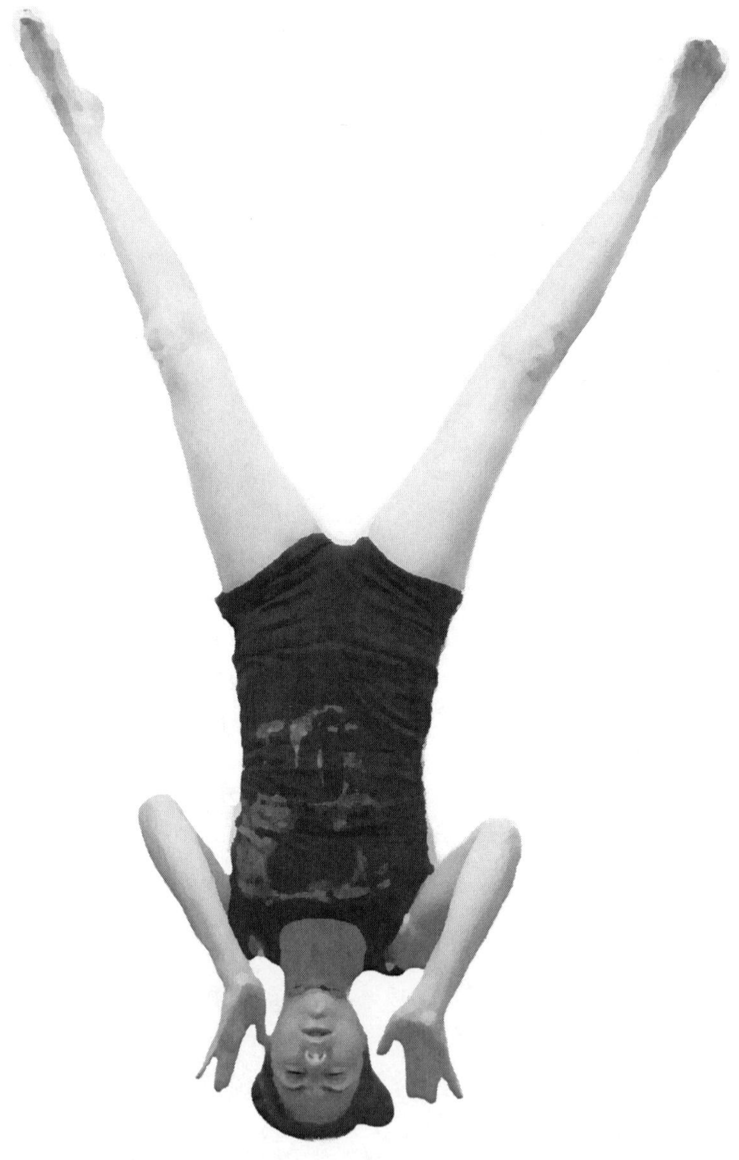

Reaching

Ok who mentions *that this* is practice?
Nooooo - *this* is not practice.
Unless all is my practice - I.e. my doctor's practice - all is my domain.
This is as it is.
Be.
This is not (about) improvement.
Improvement is not The goal.
I am not practicing my spirituality or enlightenment Here.
Here here.
Perhaps one is better off closing *this* book and practicing a head stand?
Do you think so?
Do you think?
Do I think?1
Why would you want to practice a headstand?
Can you do a headstand now? Or be in the position of a headstand? Or be with your head and forearms on the ground with 1 leg raised?
Well done. Is *this* fun?!

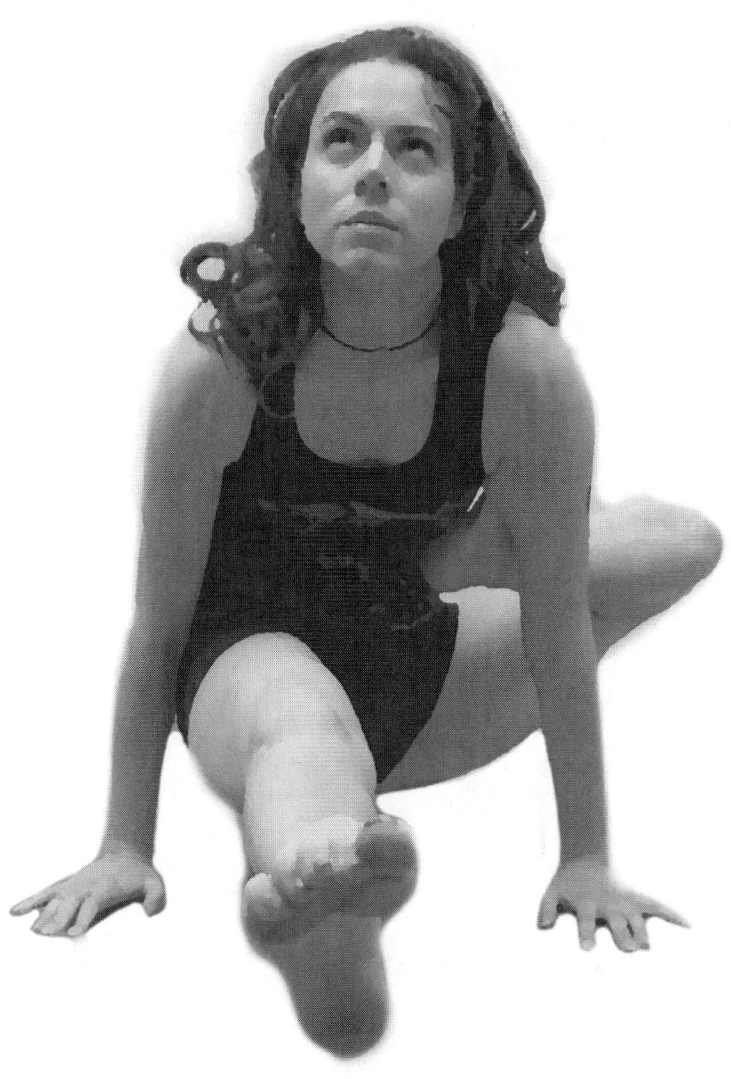

You know everything

ii) There is only me.

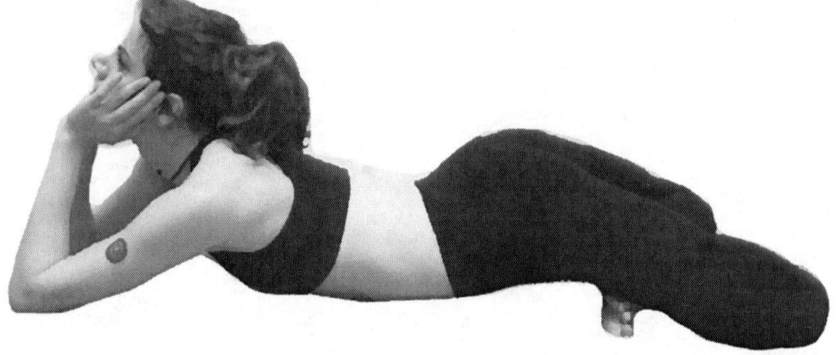

You know everything

iii) The sense of learning is not real.

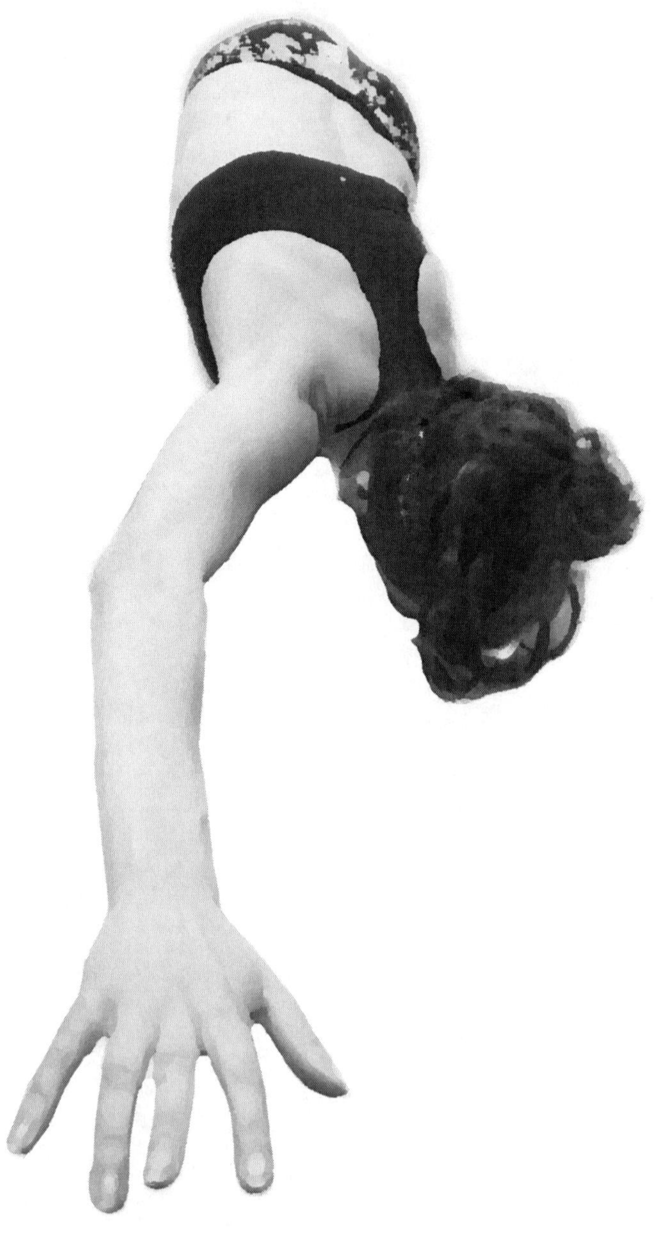

Remember nothingness.
Understand feelings, senses, thoughts and perceptions.
This collection might be one's only existence?
Let it all go.
Is there anything left?
Am I *This* word?
Only.

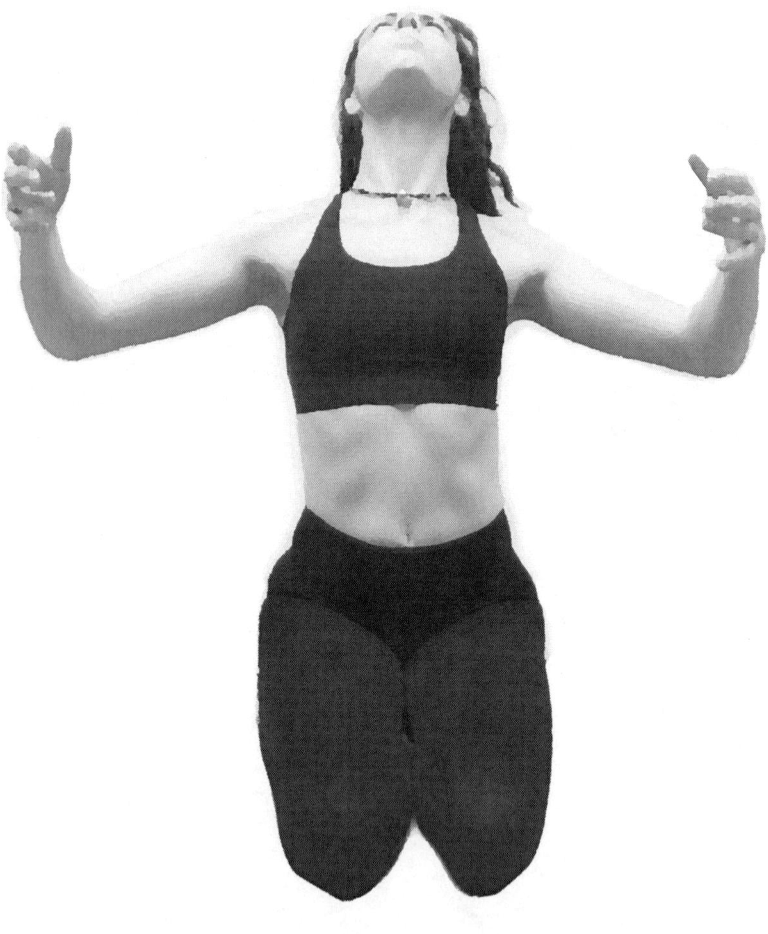

Koan

Be a know ALL.

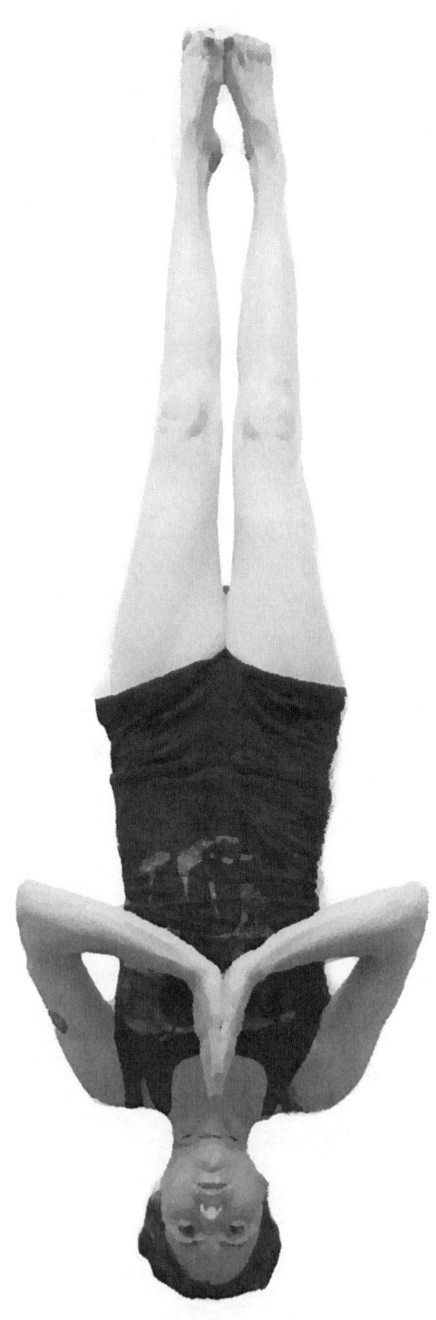

Ok inversions -
Get *This* ?!

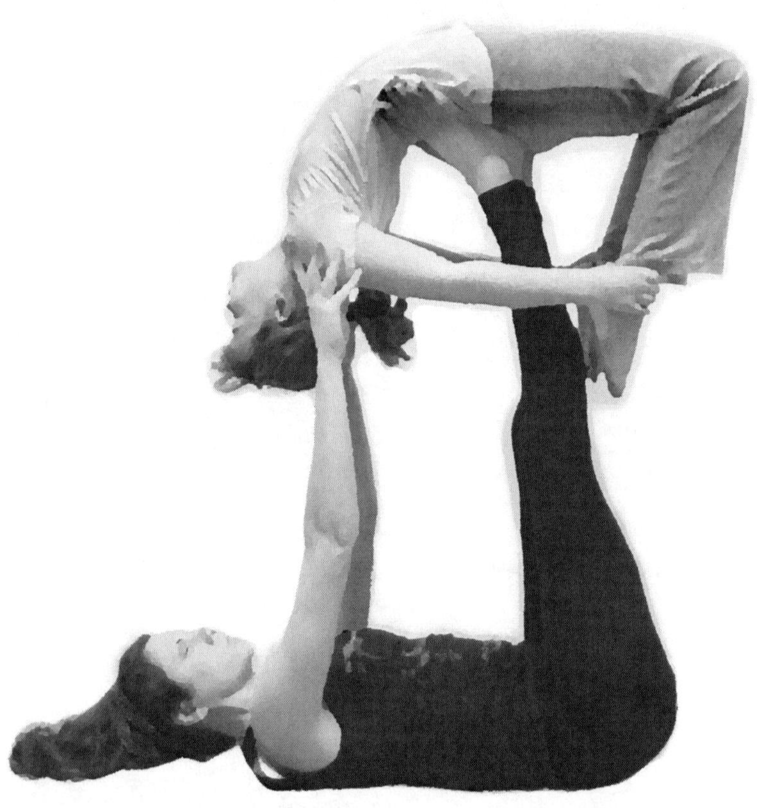

Get It?
There is only Now.
There is no one *that* teaches.
There is no learner.
There is no I teach you X + Y.

There is no doer in *this* CYoga class.

All credit is mine.
Ta.
I didn't do anything.
Get the essence.
Be the es-sence.
The essence is *this*.
This sense is sense.

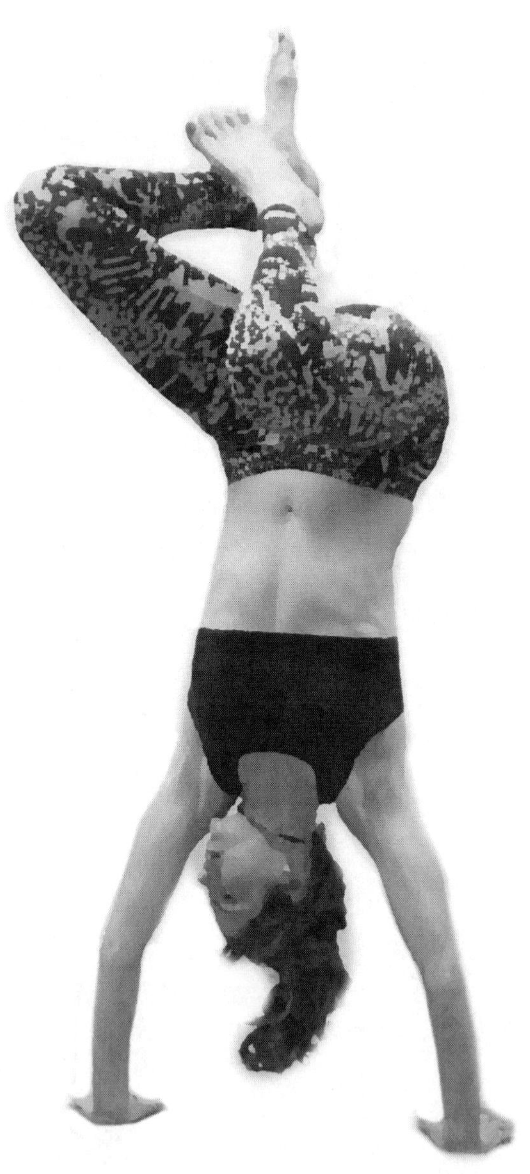

This is my first handstand!
Yes it is natural and graceful
And I am reading *this* now with the same consummate skill - with no practice.

See?
One is just here!
How one gets Here is simple.
How one gets It is\simple.
There is only *this*.

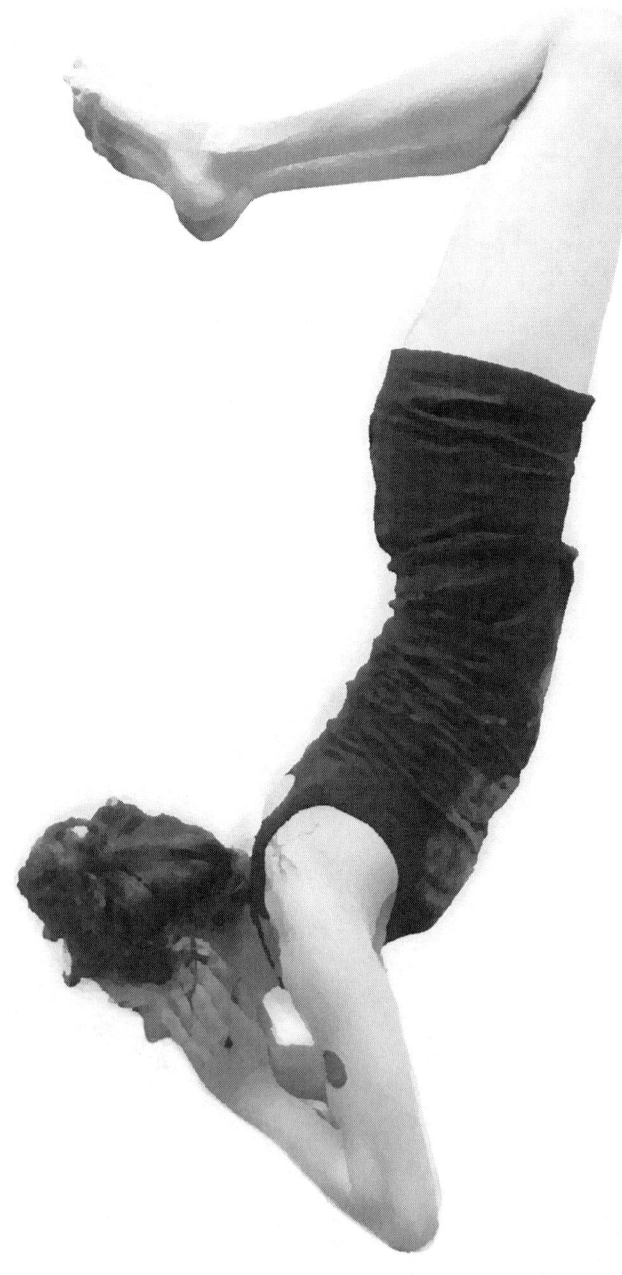

As one is everyone it is possible *that* a new born knows everything.
Born into *this* with nothing to do.
Born into *this* with nothing to accomplish.
Born into *this* with everything.
Born into *this* with no ownership.
Born and free.
How simple is *that*?

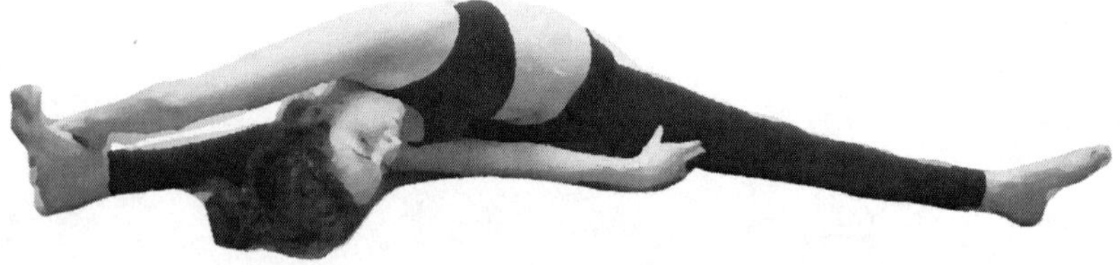

Who is I?
Who are you?
Is there only we?

Is there any them?

Forget it.
I don't care.
Do you want sex with me?

What was the 1st question?

Do you remember?

So I have your full attention.
Now I'm undressing.
How sexy is *this*?!
This is It.

Yeah enlightenment can be cool.

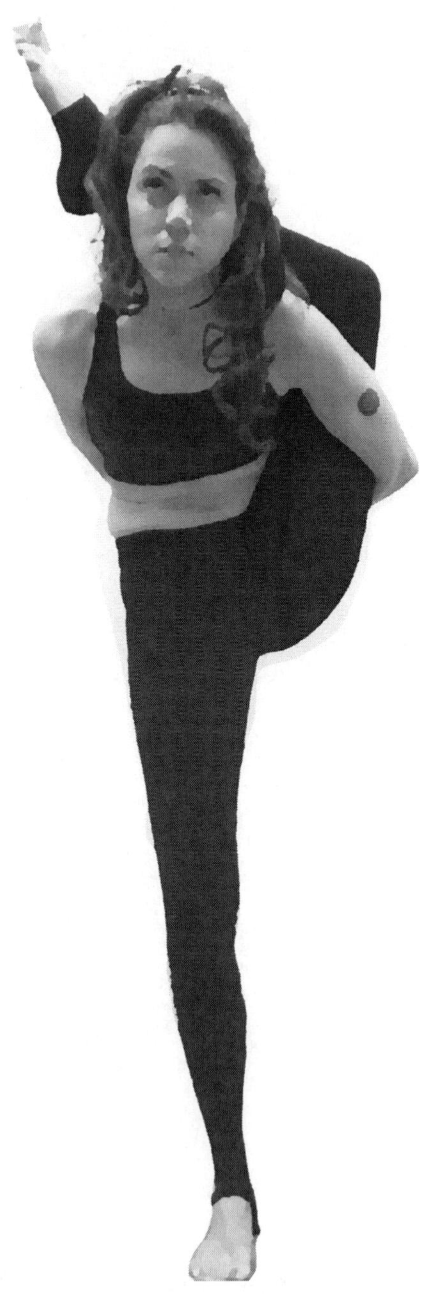

Understand Maya.
Understand *this* body.
Get anything is possible.

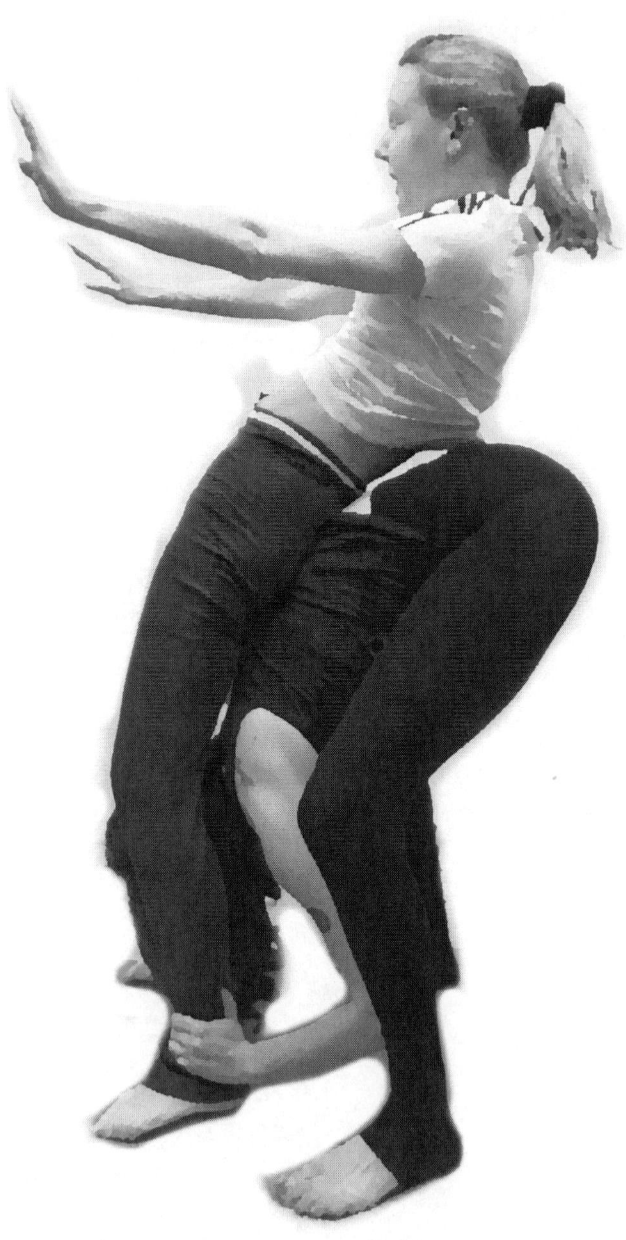

If I tell you something does *that* make two?

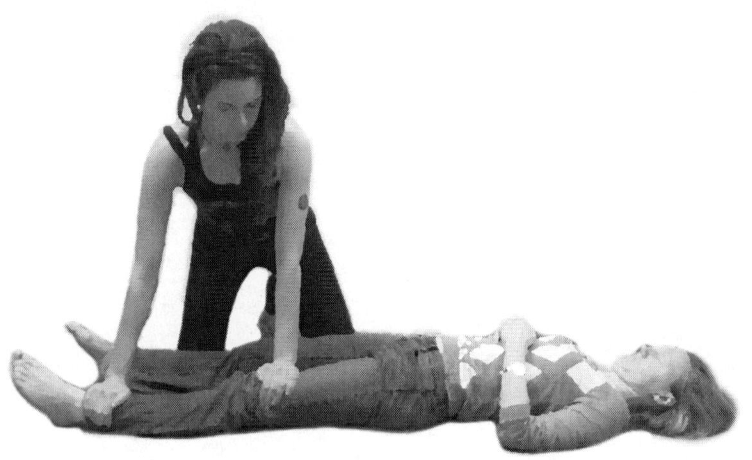

Yoga is *this* - get it?

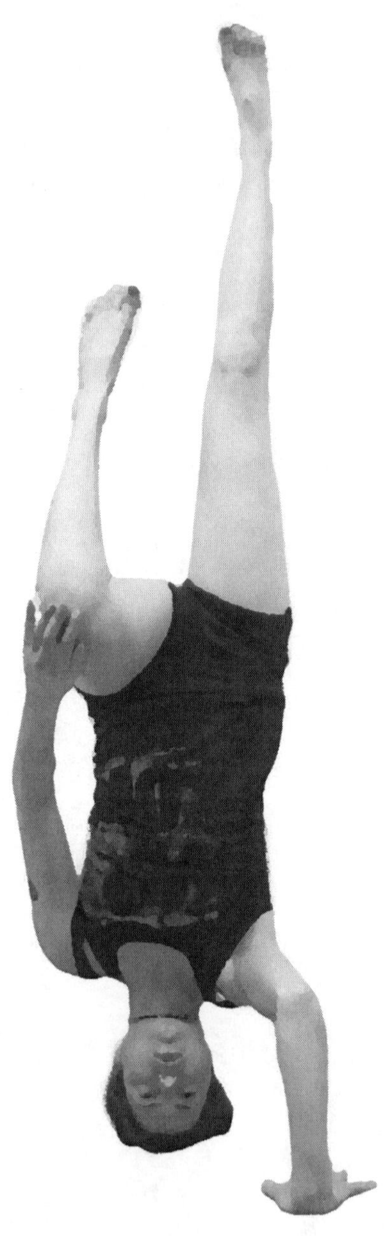

The Headstand (Sirasana)

In a headstand the brain has ample nutrients and the lymph system is relaxed.

How do you feel about the headstand? If anything.

Does my brain have enough nutrients now? Am I in a headstand?

Does my lymph system need a rest now?

Are you in a headstand now?

Do you want to be in one now?!

What about during your next yoga practice? (trick question)

Does information on benefits to yoga asanas benefit one in any way now?

What if I tell you *that* up dog and down dog are detrimental to health and ones with hernias should not do them?

Ok I make *this* up now.

See!

Do you know what a hernia is?
How could it be affected by an up dog?
Make up a way now.

Ok those with hernias should probably avoid peacock.

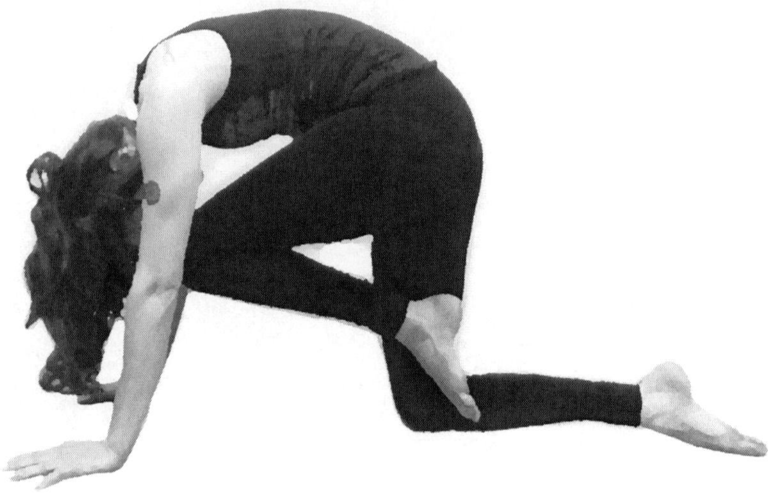

Is *this* made up now?

Do you have a hernia?

Is any of *this* relevant to your current position?

Understand *this* and oneness?!

Does *this* seem advanced yoga or very simple.

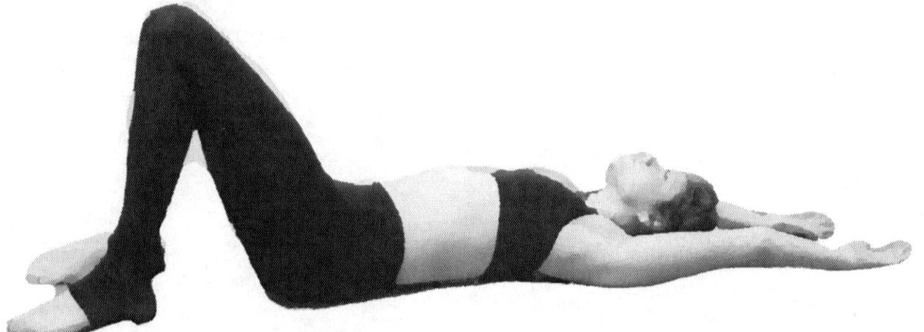

Q -What came first the chicken or the egg?

A - A circle is complete.
Join up the dots and get a circle.

Play The *This* Is It game.

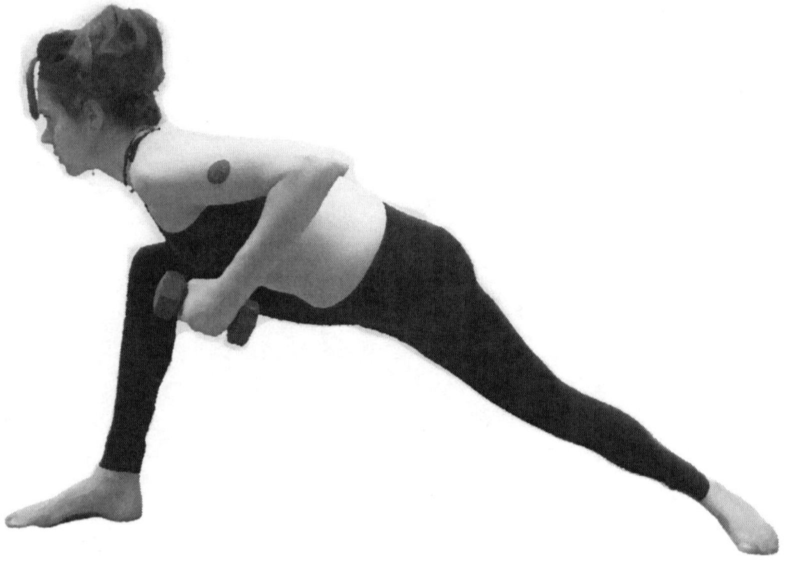

Active exercise -

Grab those dumbbells. Now put them down.
(I play on words. Are bells dumb or perhaps someone called bel is dumb?)

Ok take pen and paper. Are you with me?

If not turn the page as a yoga image presents.

If yes write a sentence on a dumbbell. Just one sentence.

i.e. The dumbbells are heavy.

Did you write it?
If yes well done.
If no write one sentence. Ok if without a pen speak one sentence on a dumbbell.
"One sentence on a dumbbell" is good enough.

Is *this* exercise done? Do you promise?

By the way when was the last moment you saw a dumbbell?
(See *This* is It Game??)

To discover the reason for *this* exercise email the sentence to:
It Is all for *this*@lycos.com.

Yes a one armed handstand is attainable by all.
See one.

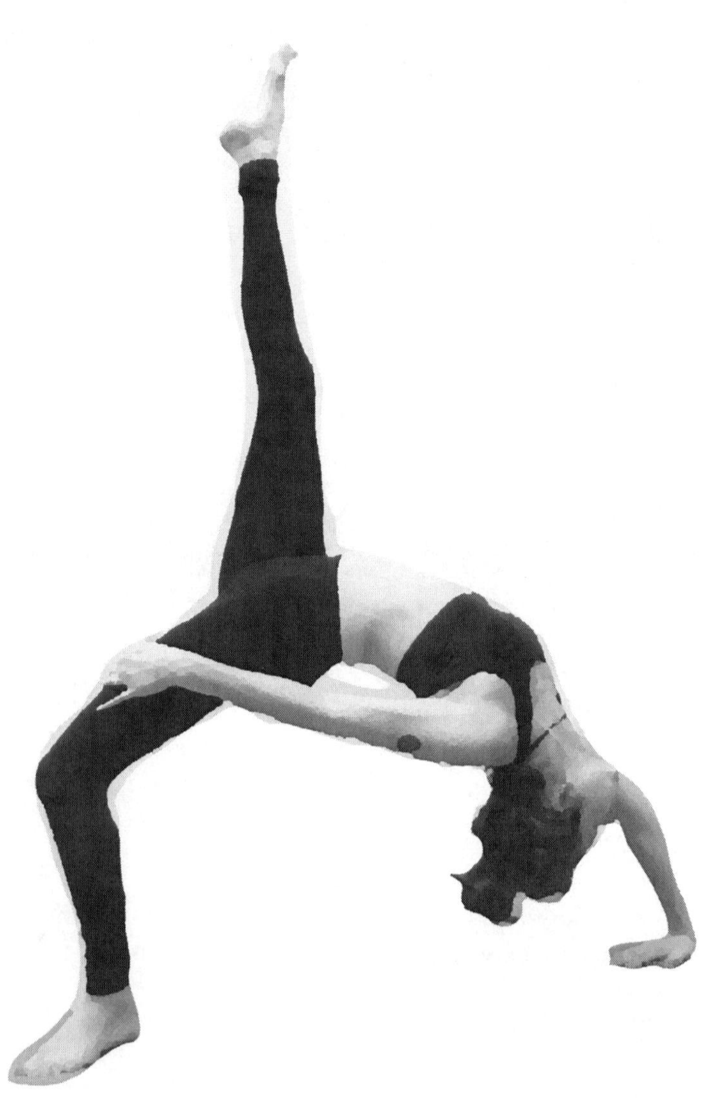

This (book) can have a dynamic interactive approach. *This* allows the manifestation of the teacher in everyone's presence.

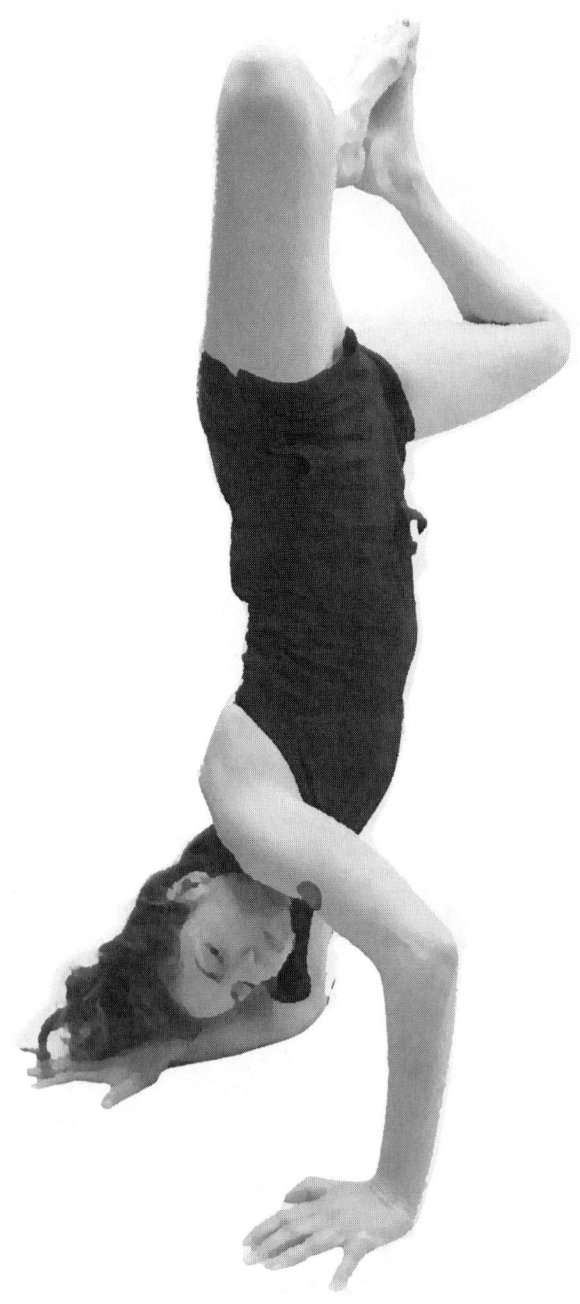

If there is a question - I .

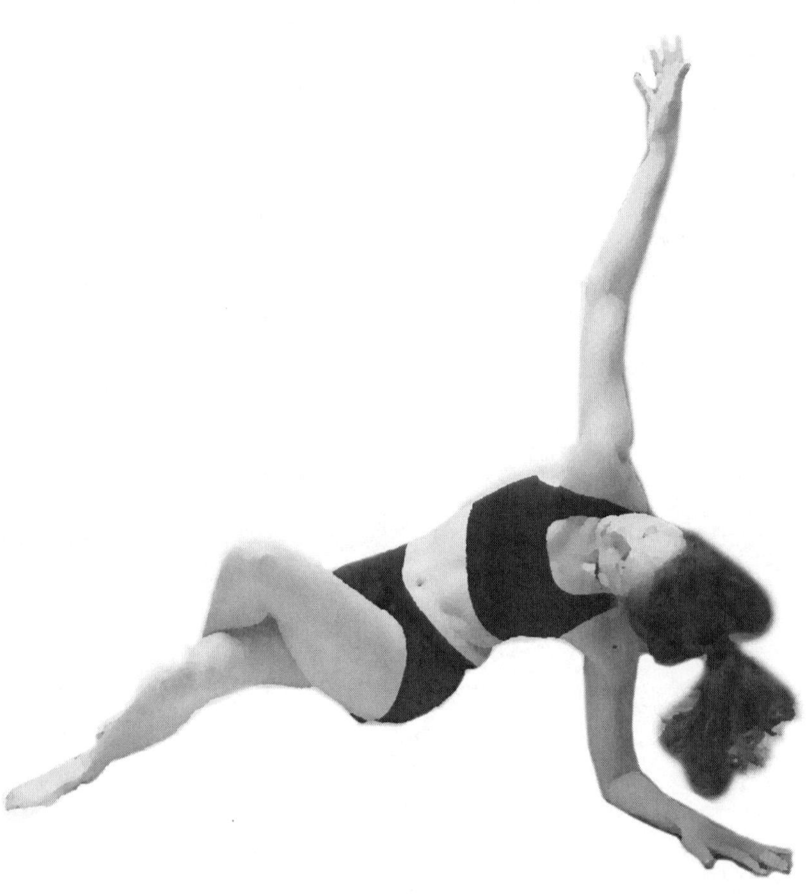

The Core (can't resist - see picture!)

A strong core can provide support for physical asanas. It is softness with strength *that* can go beyond posturing. Plank (footnote 2), sit ups, leg raises from the core can utilise and build core strength and essential awareness of core connections. Peacock is consistent with *this* allowing soft internal organs.
If possible let go of muscular tension. A strong core if present can assist effortless presence.

Play in plank with the hand pushing into the ground. Perhaps sense the grounds resistance pushing back and/or the grounds perspective allowing the I a transforming form. Allow the shoulders and deltoids integration from the straight arm into the back, rhomboids and back heart region. *This* ensures there is no collapse in the rib cage.

Placing the attention Here strength is not an issue.
Positions such as plank and shifting into up dog and down dog from the core can utilise *this* strength with the confidence of a natural uplifted position. *This* position has grace. Would you describe a graceful position as one *that* requires more or less strength and/or one *that* is at ease in the Here and Now?

A tip - keep the chest broad. Feel the serratus anterior muscles and wide lats - relax in their support and width. *This* maintains the vertical lines.
One's/ My/ *This* core is invincible.

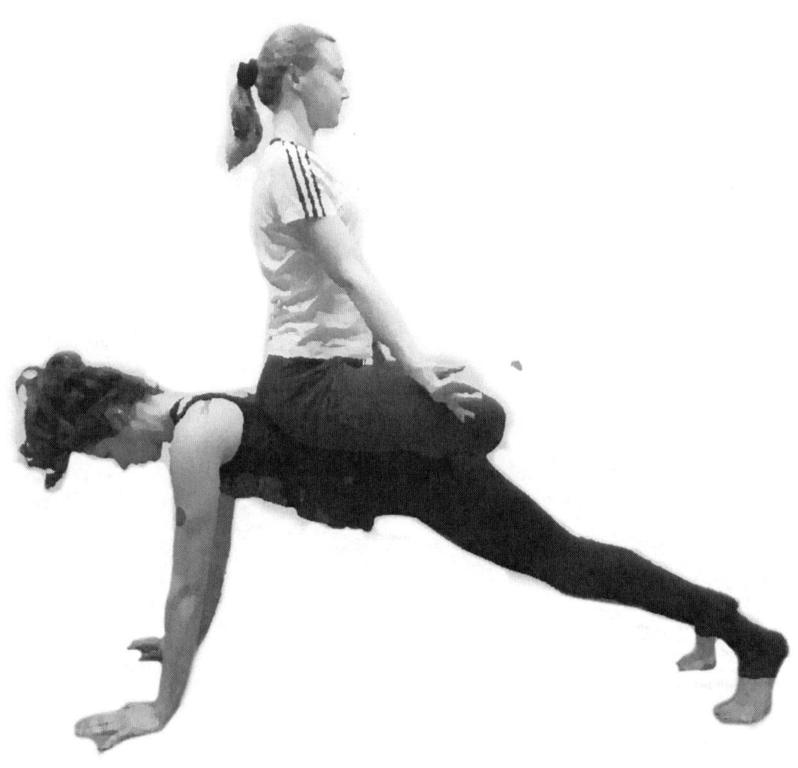

Ok about *that* - if it's not the experience I wouldn't worry about it. The experience on one level is not important.
However realise *this* experience is one's only frame of reference - ones only existence.
See *that*!
See/ be the space in *that* without buying (int(w)o) anything.
That includes me.

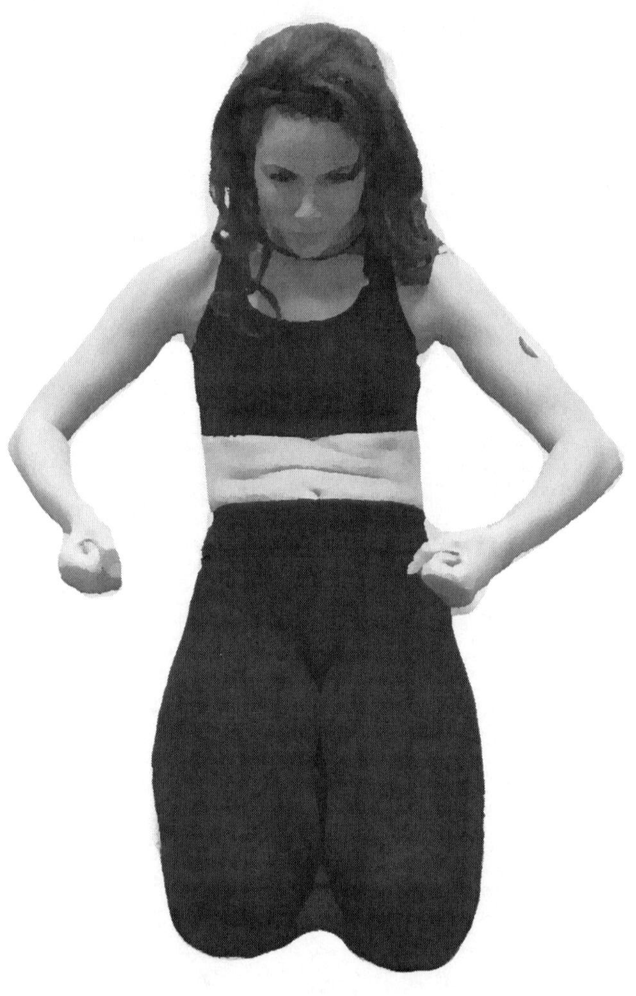

Energy/ Prana/ Chi/ Om/ Now

energy - whatever it is - if more than a word - is here now (energy!)

the idea of being or doing something not now can accompany a sense of where is the energy? see1

yes i always am energy - if i create it .

that is the beauty of cyoga.

it is all now -

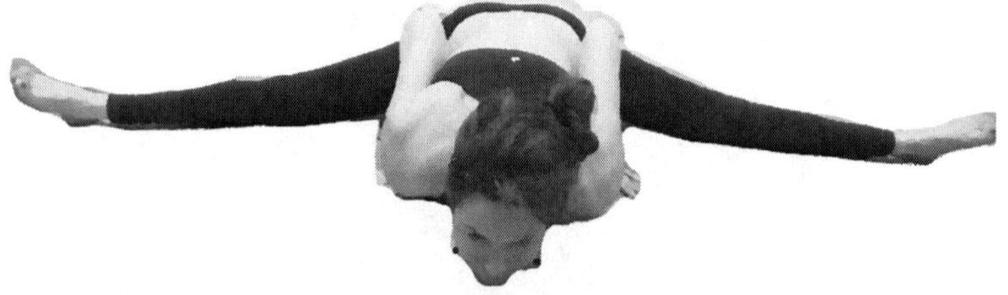

Beginners excitement

It is for everyone.
It can be exciting.
Yippeeeee.

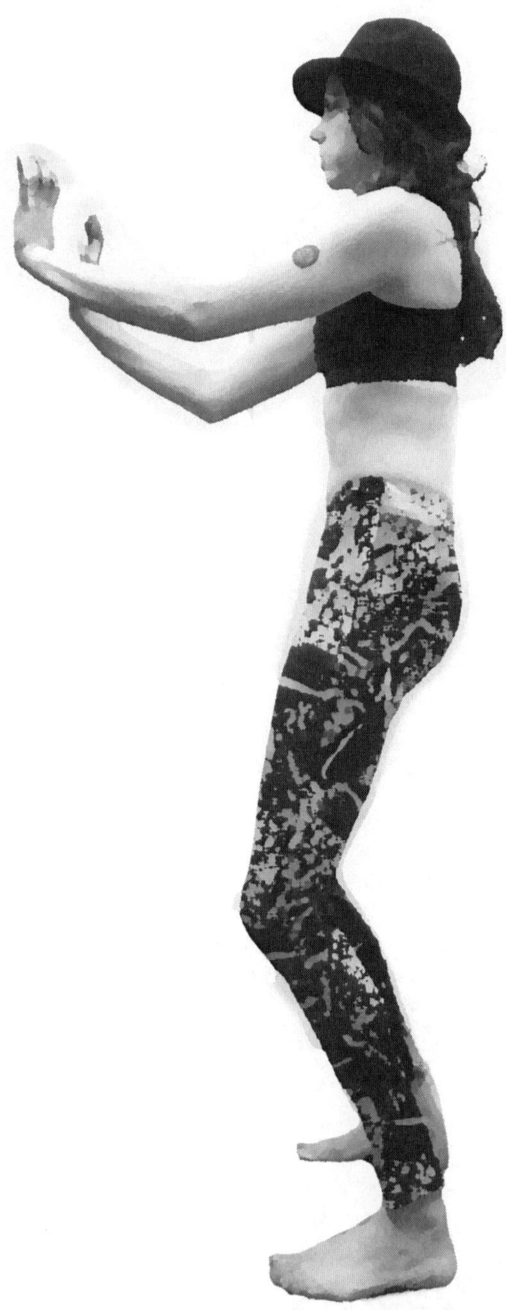

Nutrition

Are you eating?
Really it is very simple
Eat what you want.
How much can you eat now?
Just *this*!

Ay organic is good. My meaning is sooo simple. It includes saying no to GM and chemical pesticides.

Oh well.

Is now a good moment to mention Maya.

Ok don't eat apples
Are you eating an apple now?
So - don't worry about it.
Ok you can eat apples - see the point.

Can one can eat but not eat?
See nothing is special.

I - eat what you/ I want.
If you/ I understand you/I may not eat at all.
Am I eating now?

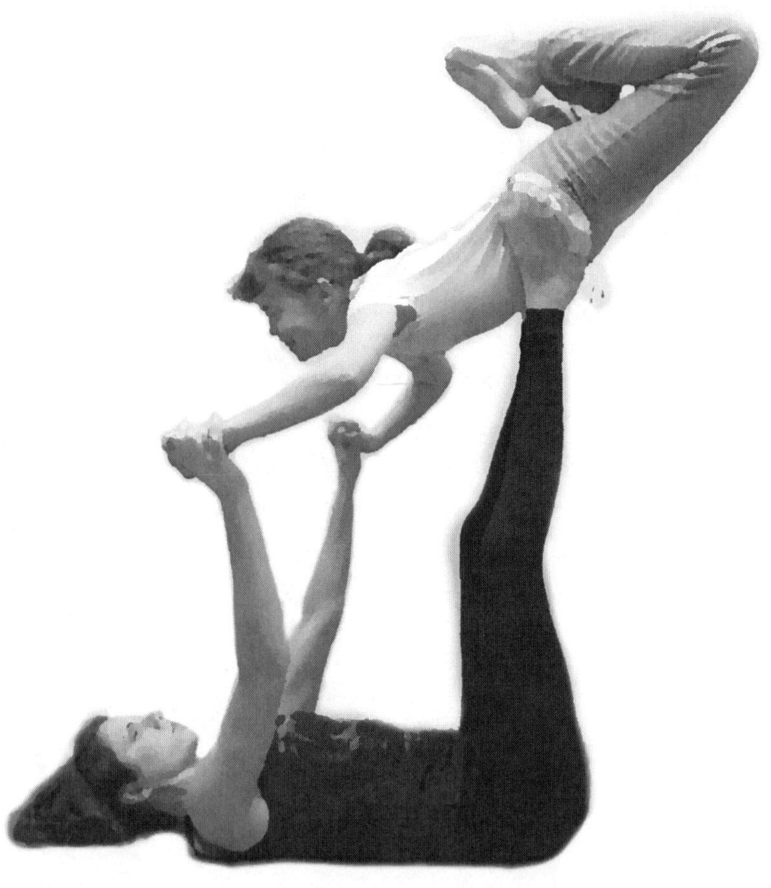

Savasana

Exhale and feel the diaphragm relax. Is there a sense of relaxation *that* permeates the whole body?

Relax the sides of the nose.
Relax the cheekbones.
Relax the upper palate.
Relax the lower palate.
Relax the scalp.
Relax the ears.
Relax the jaw.

Feel any heaviness in the body.
Allow *this*. Drop it. I ground. Become one with the ground. Be the ground.
Feel nothing.
There is no body.

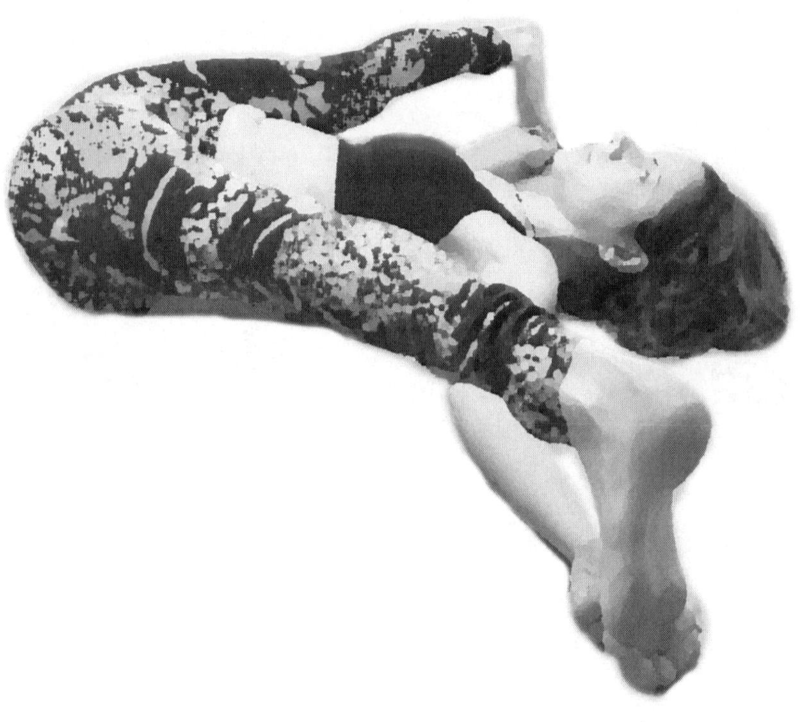

Does the fact *that* I am adept at posturing with no practice appear magnanimous?

Cool - huh!

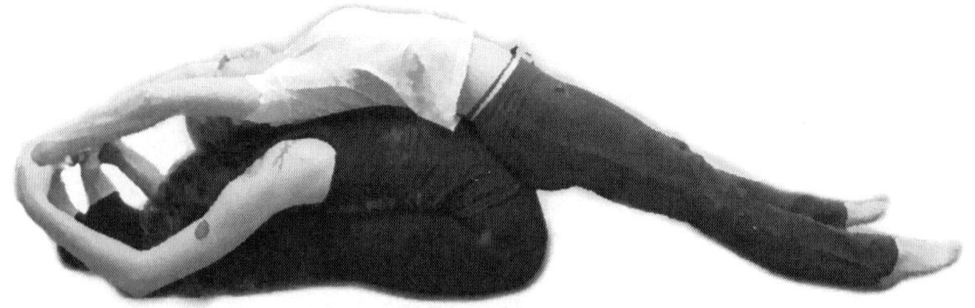

With all the good intentions *This* Is It!
This is A1.

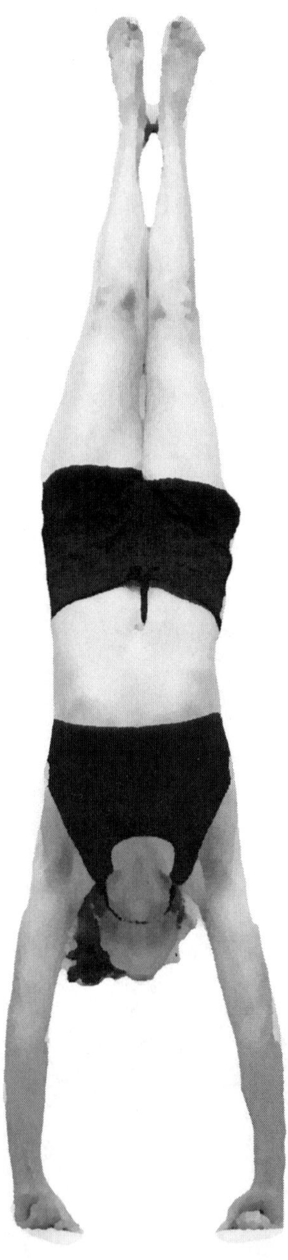

There are no favors.

(Why?
Answer - see *This* is It Game)

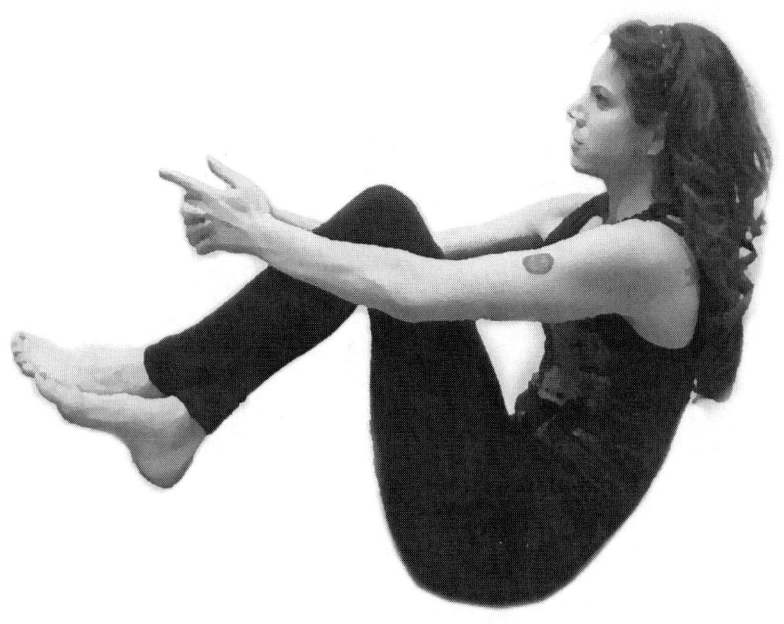

One is still always - however it may appear.

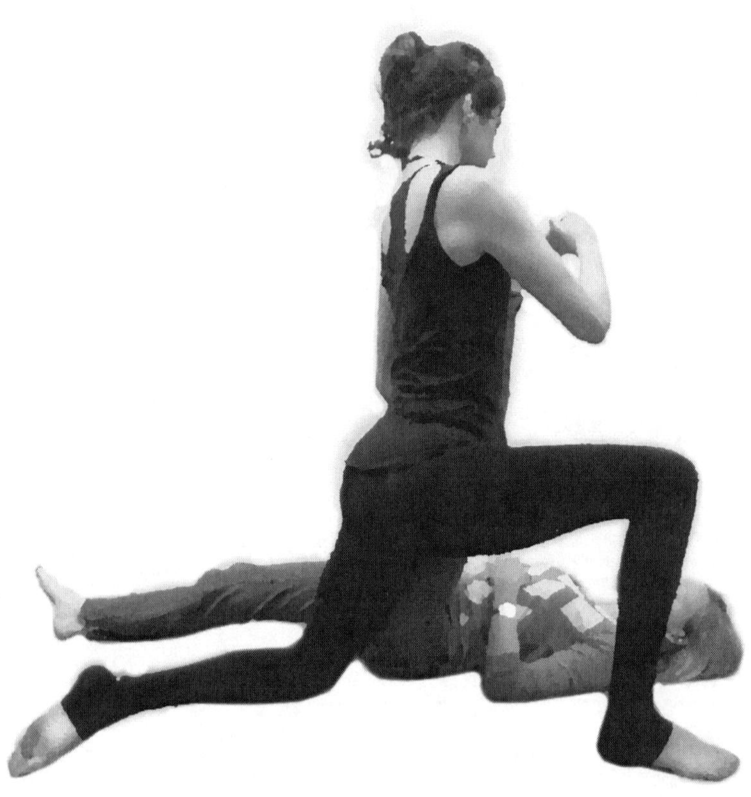

Meditation Retreat?

When are we going?!

(*This* is It game)

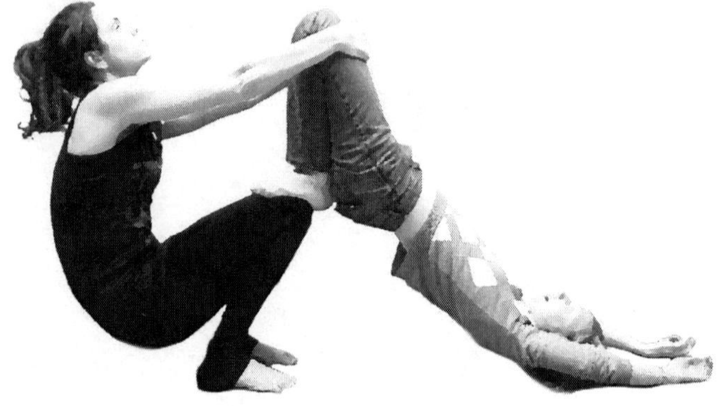

Is there is a sense of improvement or goal setting? *This* is (a) sense.

There is no special sense.

Improvement is Maya.

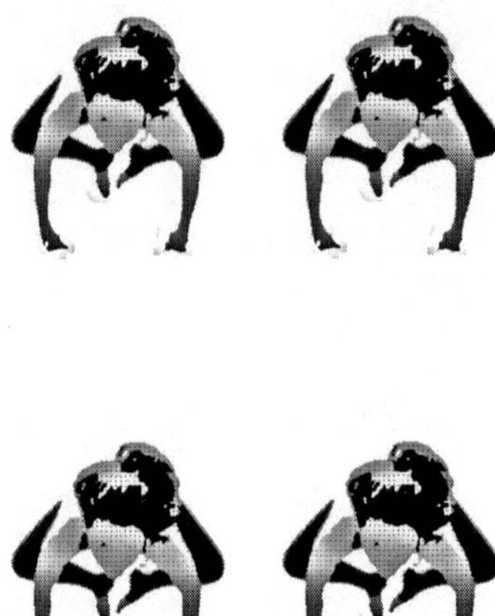

Discipline

There is no discipline involved in *This*.
I am the winner!
Yes I am born as a perfect headstand.
I am serious.
Can one understand *that*?!
A feat, if it exists, is not special.
The position I am now, always, is not the result of discipline.
I am no disciple.
This is born now - it is as it is.
Seeing these words is not a discipline.
This is crucial to understanding why you have achieved everything right here right now.
Your position now is effortless.
My position is now effortless.
The sense/ fact of being born now is without effort - as it is.

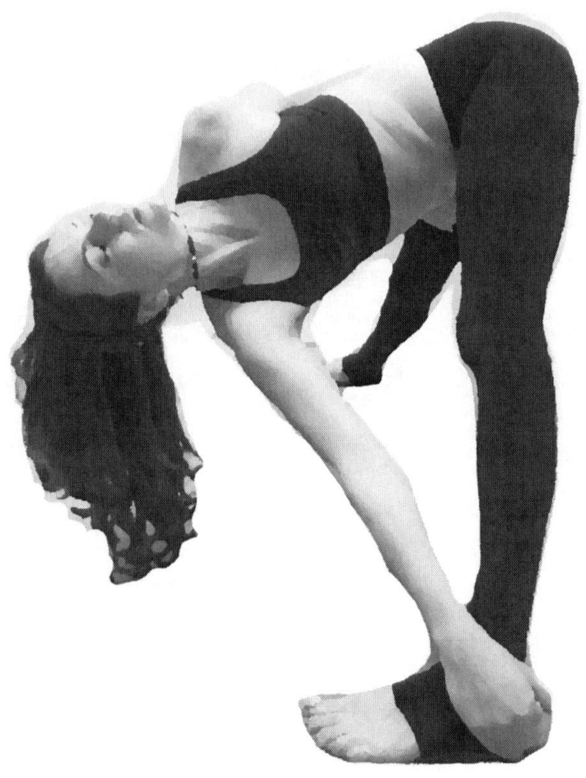

Release the shoulders

Relax the pectoralis (front of the chest), trapezius and serrratus anterior (sides of the chest).
Feel the shoulders drop .
Allow the spine between the scapulae' (shoulder blades) support.
Focus on *that.*
Let the surroundings (muscles around the spine) release and leave awareness.
Focus on one's spine.
This is one's support.

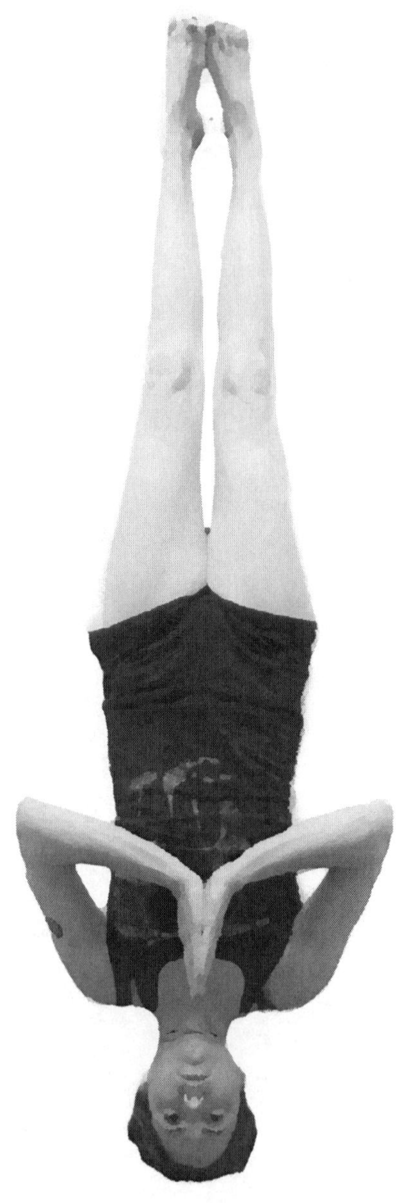

Chi

Chi is available now.
Feel the fingertips.
Feel the toes.
What is chi?
What do you feel in the fingertips and toes?
Nothing is special.

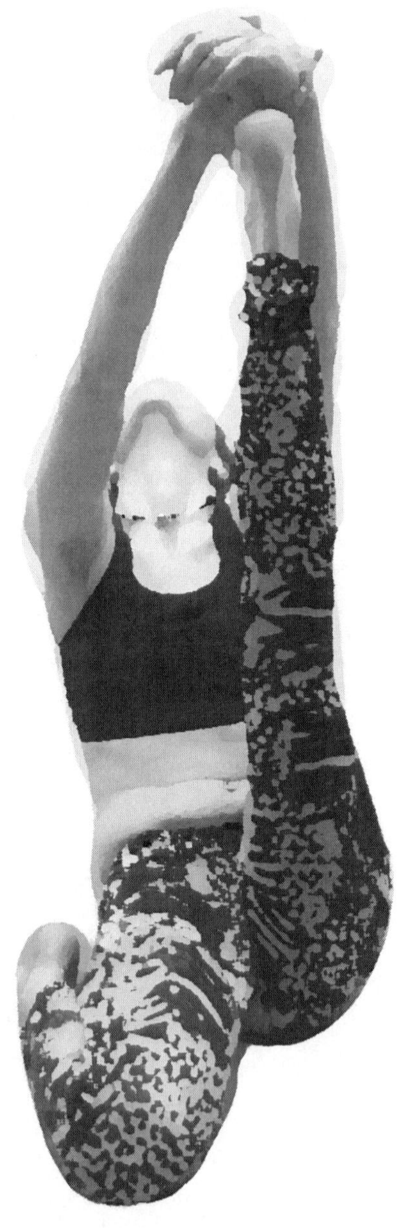

CYoga rules.

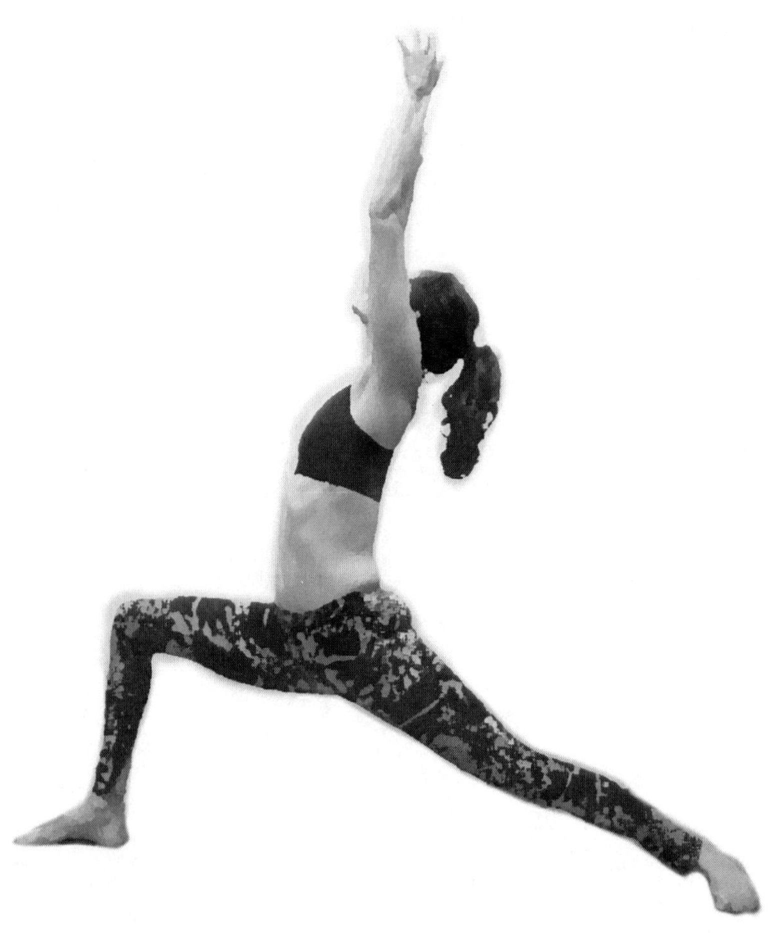

A unique softening is available Here.
Performance of an asana is
An opening to the truth
A tribute
Allow the space
There is no space between asanas
There is just space
There is no coming and going
There is no getting into and getting out of a position
There is *this* position
The space is Here
The space is available where One is.
That is Here.

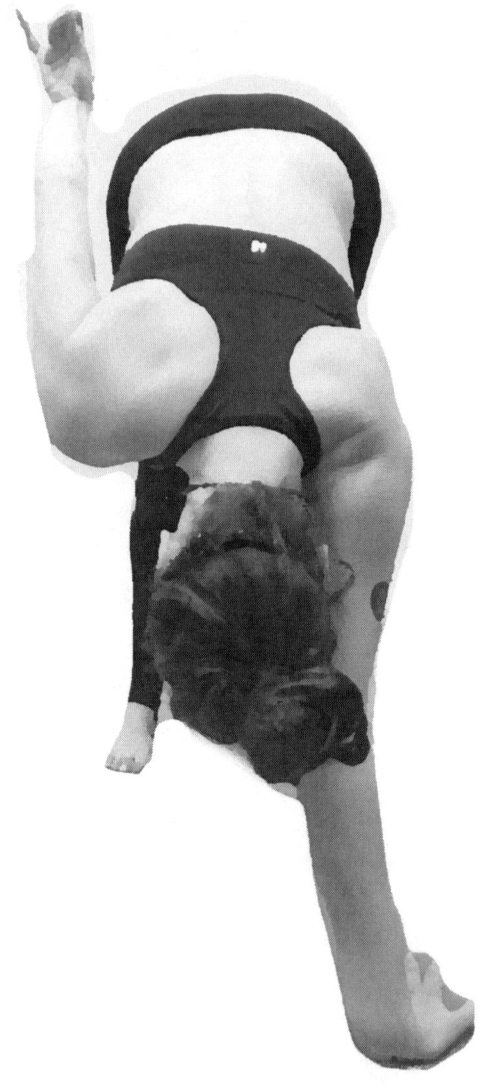

Tenesgrity

There might be a sense of tension.
There might be a sense of friction.
There might be sense of release.
Allow the effortless sense.
The effortless sense is *this* sense.
The achievement is *This*.

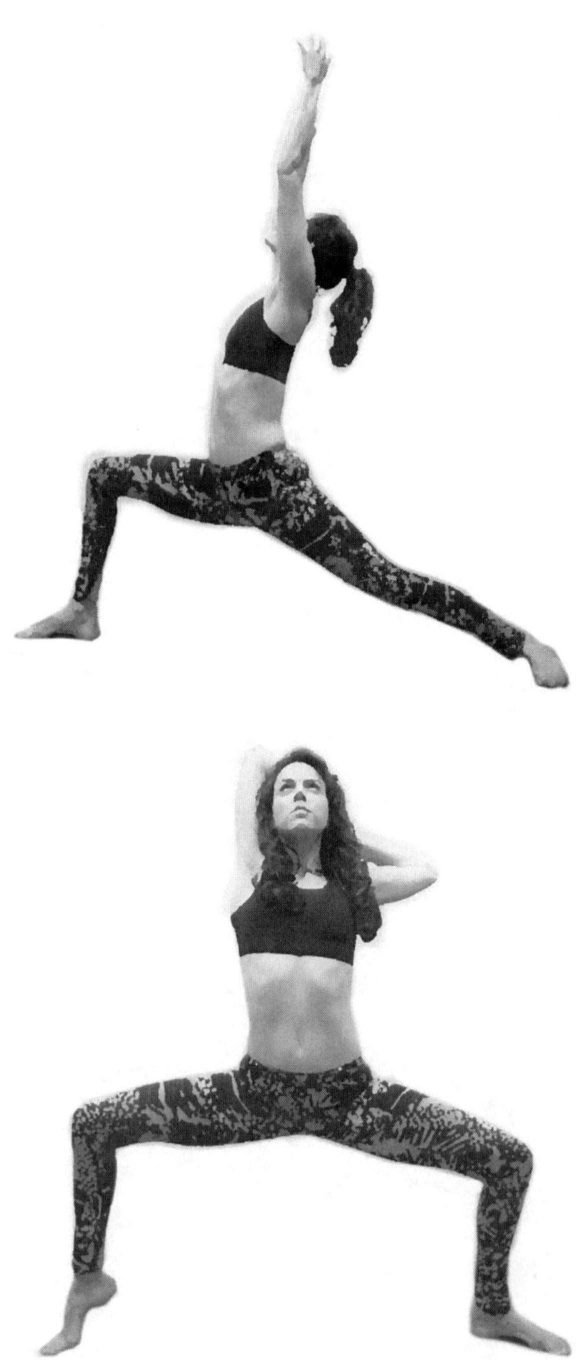

Right Now

One movement.
Playing with *This*
One movement.
Working with *This*
One movement.
This one movement
Seeing through it
There is no movement
Here Now.

Understand the sense of movement.
This is it!

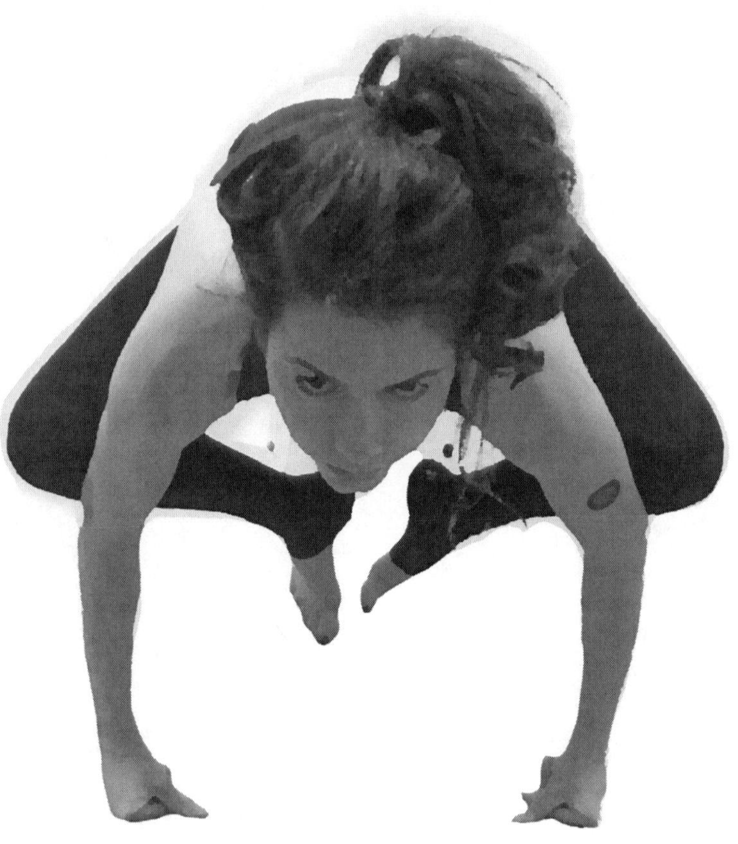

Yoga is an all body workout
Yoga can be considered exercise;
Yoga can work strength, flexibility, agility and coordination
One can mention benefits such as tight abs, cute ass, lithe body ; a great immune system; a strong skull (strong bones; perfect neurovascular system etc.

Yet from one perspective there are no benefits.
See all sides.
From *this* side the fruit of yoga is only evident in the present.
This is the greatest/ only gift one presents.
Being is the yoga is solo.
Being is the only prize.

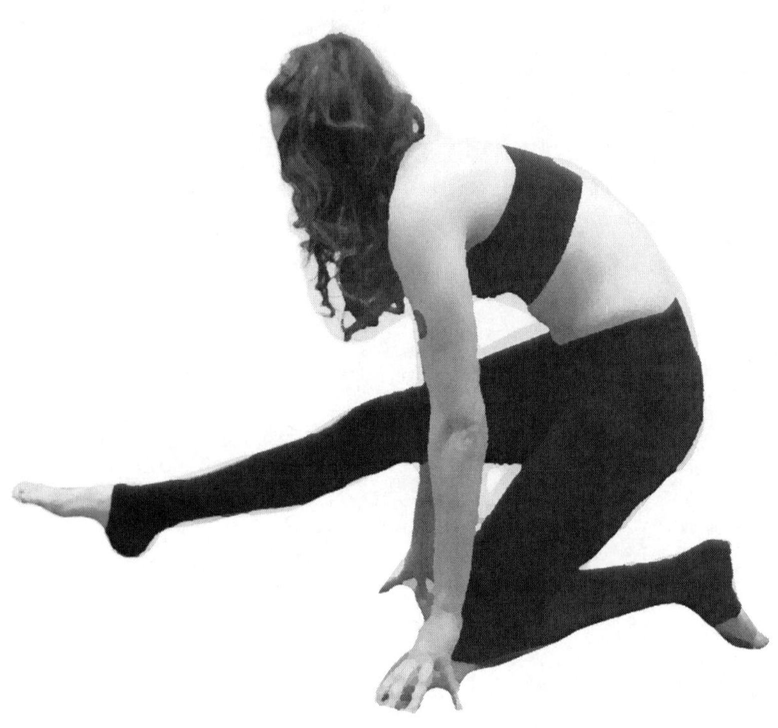

Sparring

Acute presence is created now.
Grounded, depth and ultimate victory is *this*.
The knockout in martial work is not a lack of presence.
One is always present.
Understand oneness.
Flooring is a set up.
One does not become one with an opponent/partner.
It may feel *that* way.
One is one.
Yoga is all encompassing.
One is always victor.
Flooring is a set up - now forget *this*!
Otherwise you are floored.
(No worries - if *this* is it!)

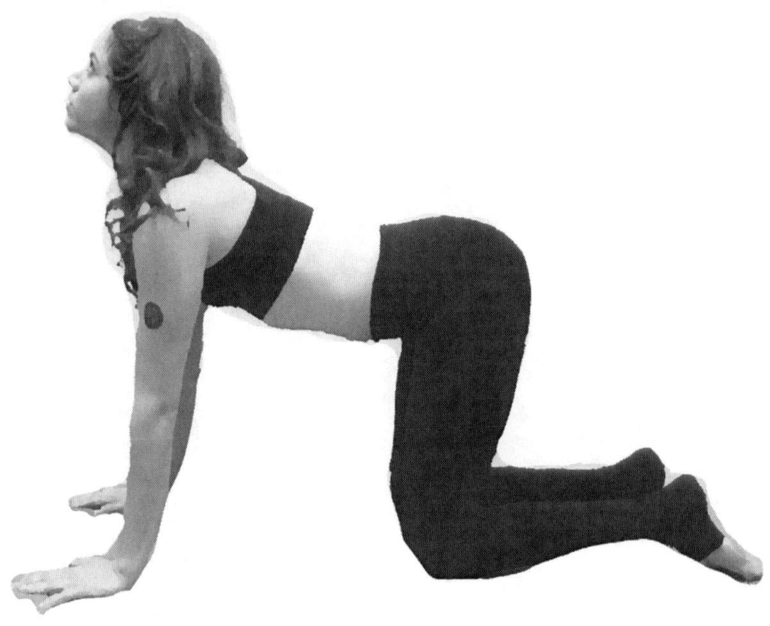

There is no Time (Ti-me)
One can create a story of someone who did *this* and *that*.
Open the sides of the eyes and see *this* page.
The whole story is Here Now.
Now focus on *THIS* word
This part of the story, I, is created now.
Or is *this* the whole story?
Is there ever rest?
Rest now.

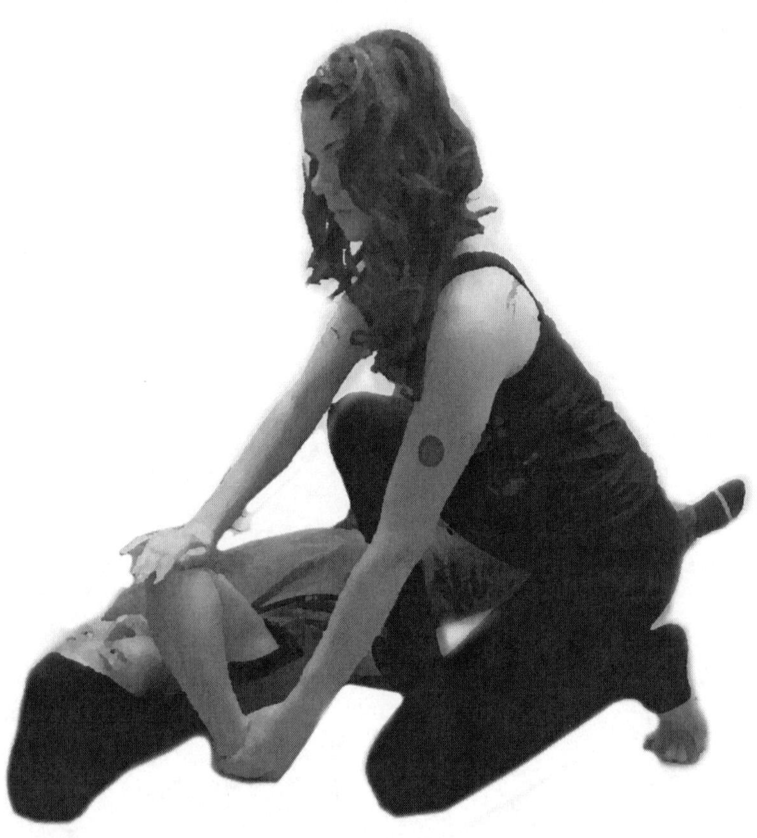

Nothing's Personal

Everything is one.
That/ this is more than interconnection or connection. There is no agenda Here Now (in *this*) - there is nothing to/2 lose and nothing to/2 gain.
Yes there is/ can be supreme bliss/ peace with *this*.
Is *that* your experience now.
Yes I am utter peace and bliss1.

There is no one is realized and another is not.
I do not care about realization.
It is me.
The concept of *this* is right.
Is the concept of restraint or observance of virtue relevant? These words are read/ created now.
Is *this* observance of my virtue?!

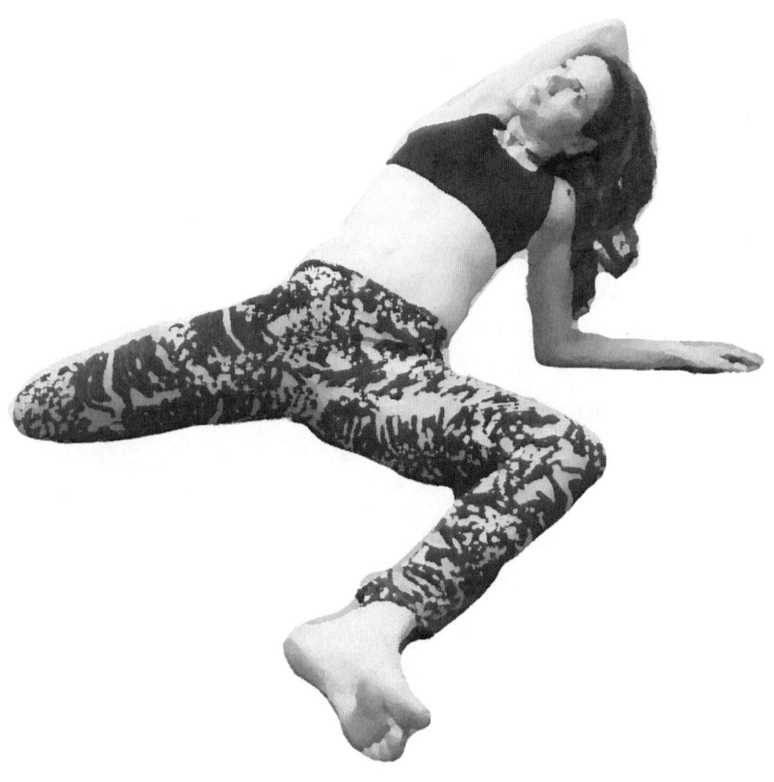

Thine Self Be True

You what?!1
There is only thy self.
What is the truth now?
Nothing is personal - is *this* sense now creating a duel of agreement or not?

Yes there is only thy self. So if i stand firm in my self what's the problem? = there isn't any.
for me anyway!

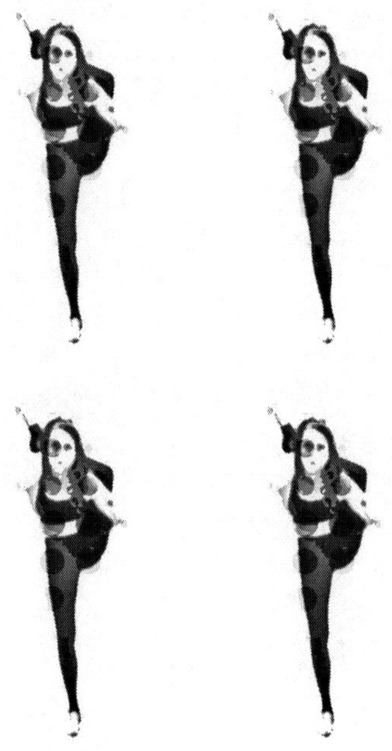

C

Rub the palms feeling ones creation.
Place the right palm over the left ear cupping it gently.
Place the left palm (or fingertips) on the floor.
Gently tilt the head to the right
Feel the neck stretch.
Feel the listening.
Possibly hear the C.
Rub the palms feeling ones creation.
Place the left palm over the right ear cupping it gently
Place the right palm (or fingertips) on the floor.
Gently tilt the head to the right.
Feel the neck stretch.
Feel the listening.
Possibly hear the C.
Rub the palms feeling ones creation.
Place the palms over the eyelids - eyes closed.
Where is the C now?

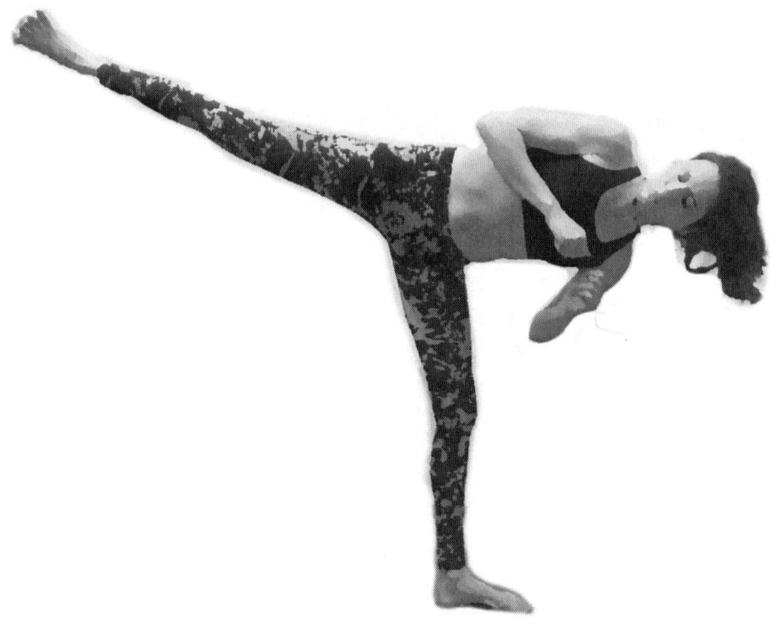

Is *this* an illusion?
That is Maya.

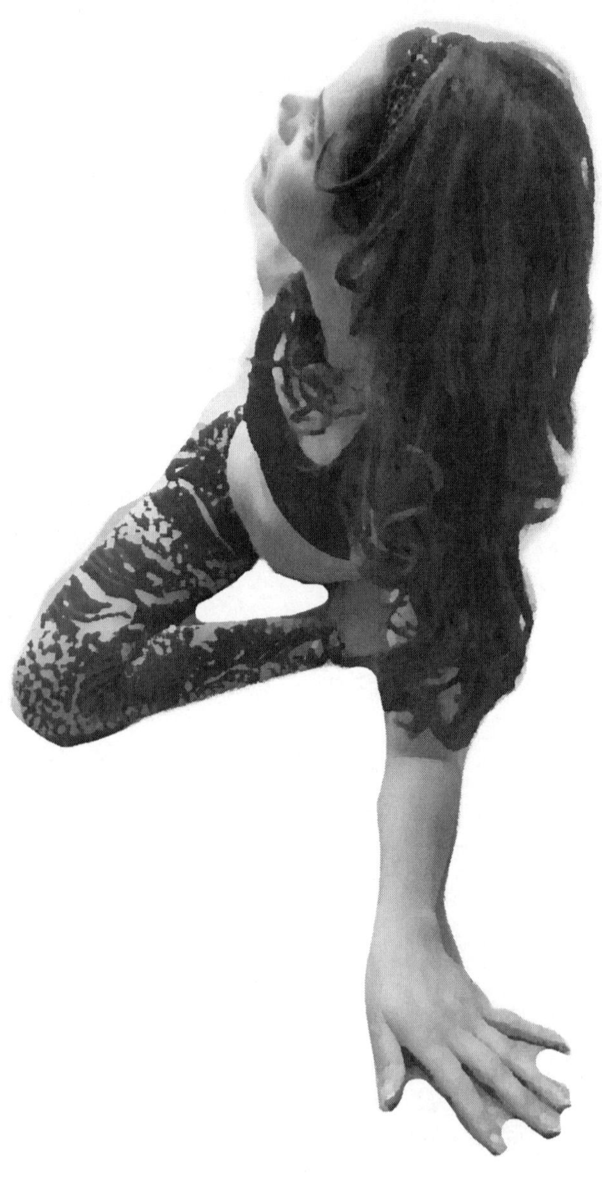

Playing with dance.
Working with martial artistry.
Seeing through yoga.

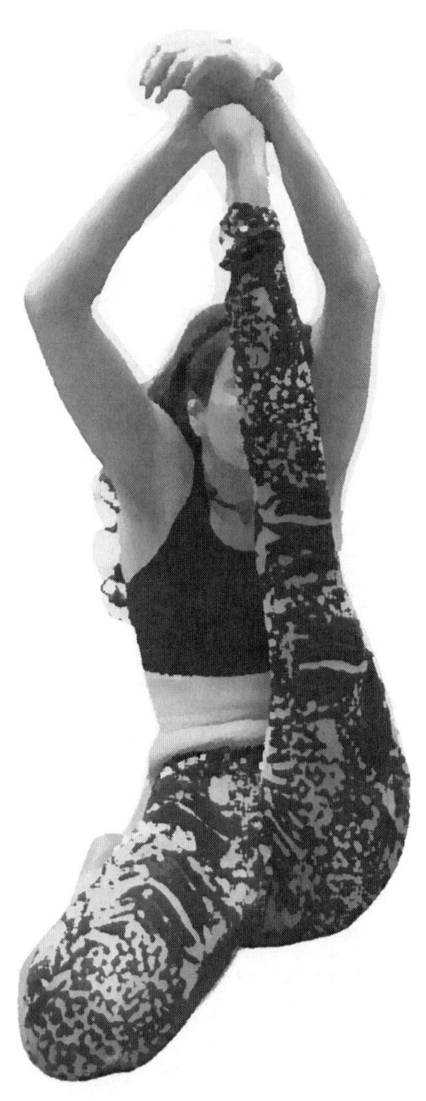

YOu Go = A

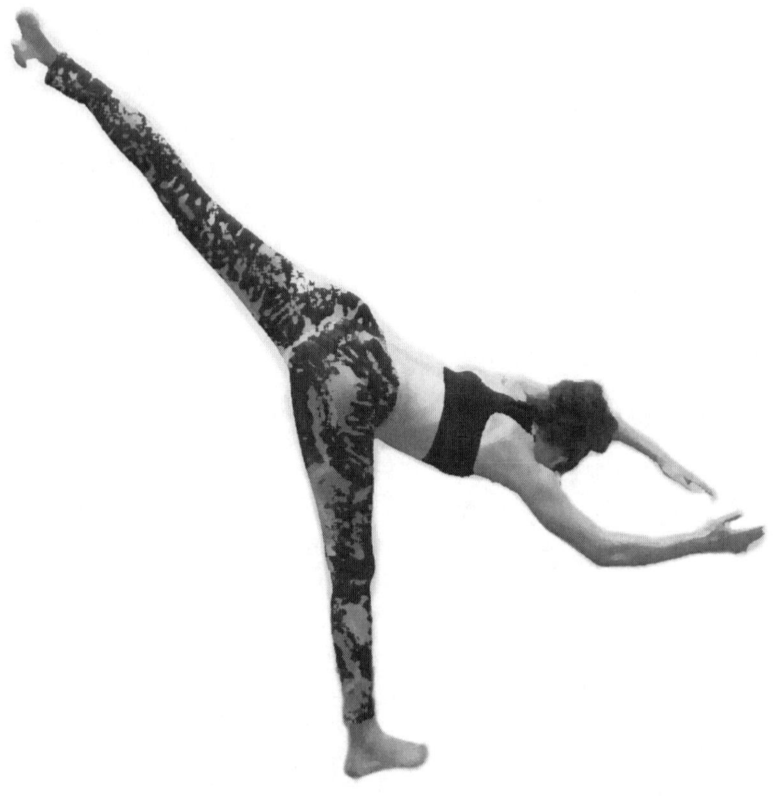

I create myself now.

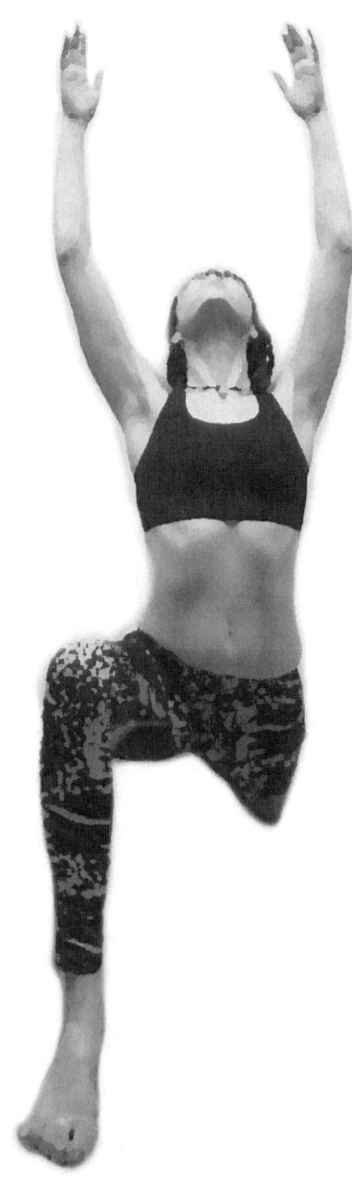

CYoga Tai Chi

Tai chi can be known as boring slow movements or grace in one movement. Ones perspective is every.

Cutting the label tai chi chuan i christen "tai chi chuan" "*this*" and "CYoga" . 2 names - cool!

so is it necessary to attend classes and practises to become master of tai chi or *this* or CYoga?

1. Forget mastery - the name master denotes an inferiority to Beauty (*that* is me). Be CYoga. Be *This*. Anyway why would anyone who has *this* experience want mastery? Rank and status are stripped in *this* light. Imagine anyone who considers/ calls themselves a master naked and see the truth. Strip the master.

2. You are/ I am right no classes or practises are necessary. One is here now. *This* is the highest attainment. Know *that* = know your/ my magnificence.

3. *This*/ CYoga is very simple.

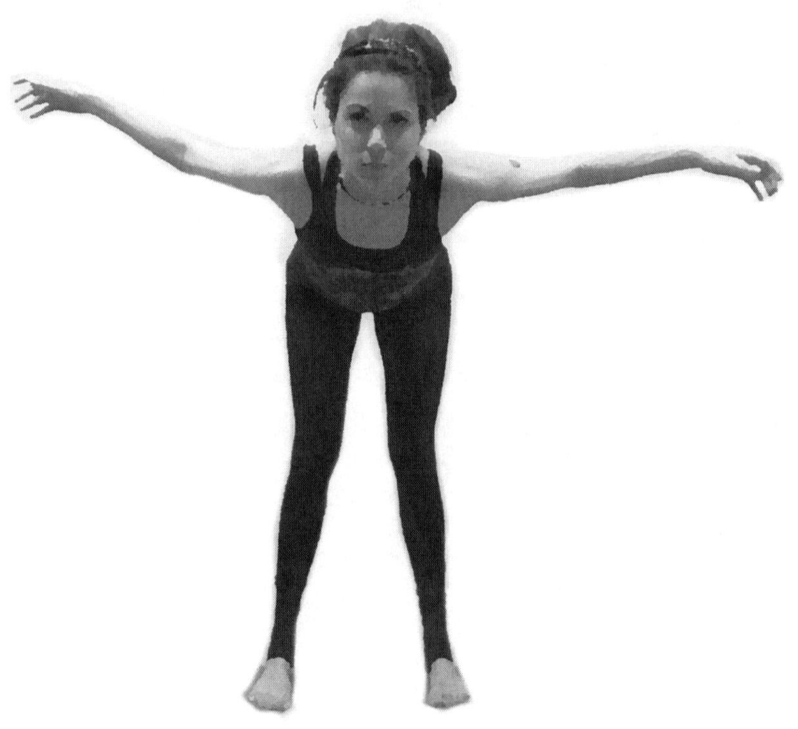

Mix it up

Make tai chi capoiera
Make capoiera at chi
Make yoga a tango
Make jujitsu jazz
Make
It happens
It works
The essence is It.
The essence is on.
The essence I s *this*.
Is there only one?!?

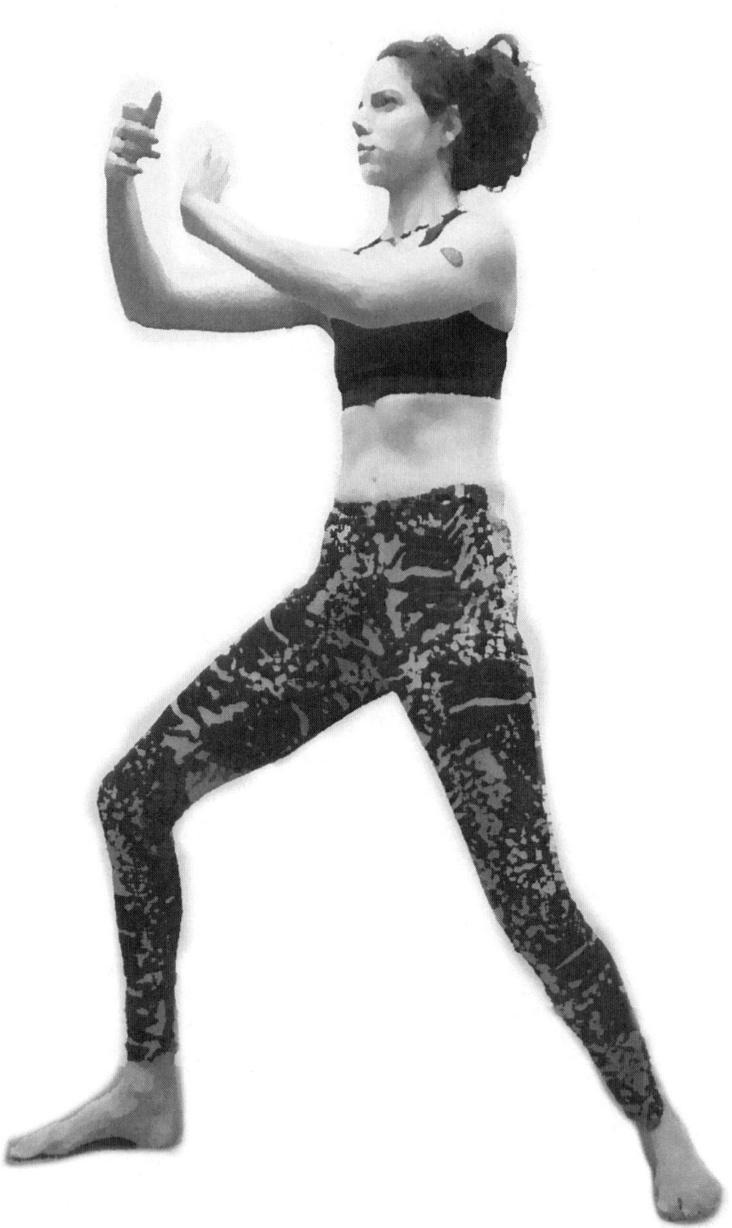

Place the tip of the tongue where the upper palate joins with the teeth ridge..
Lengthen the neck.
Feel the spine extending through the neck.
Feel peace.

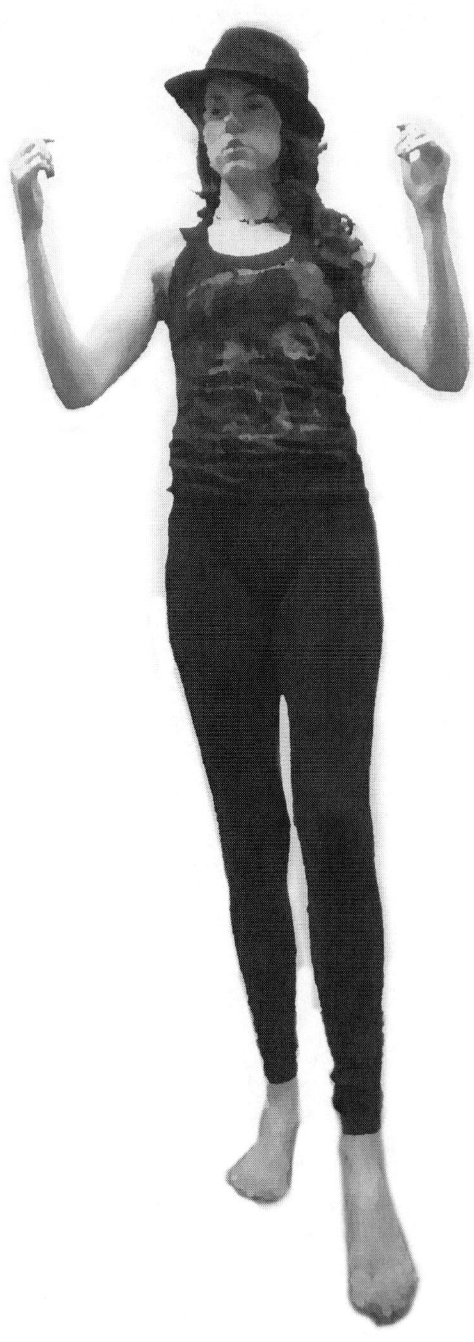

One creates *this*
inspiration is *this*

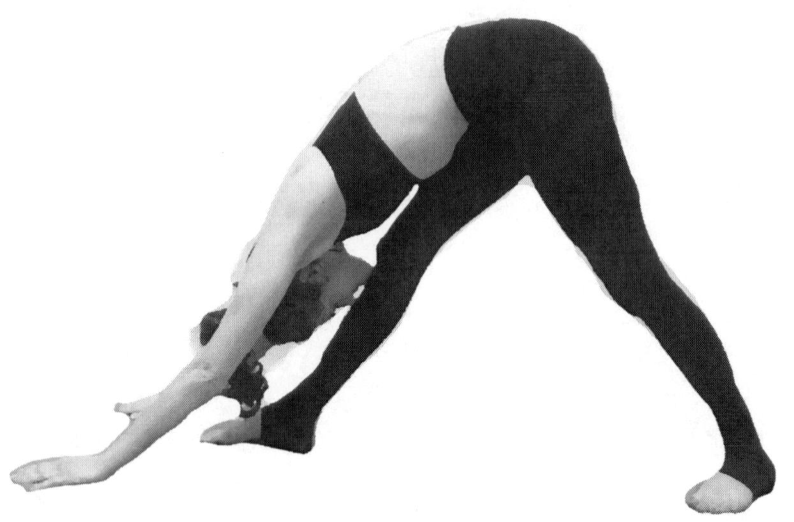

Light

This prism of light creates *this* illusion.

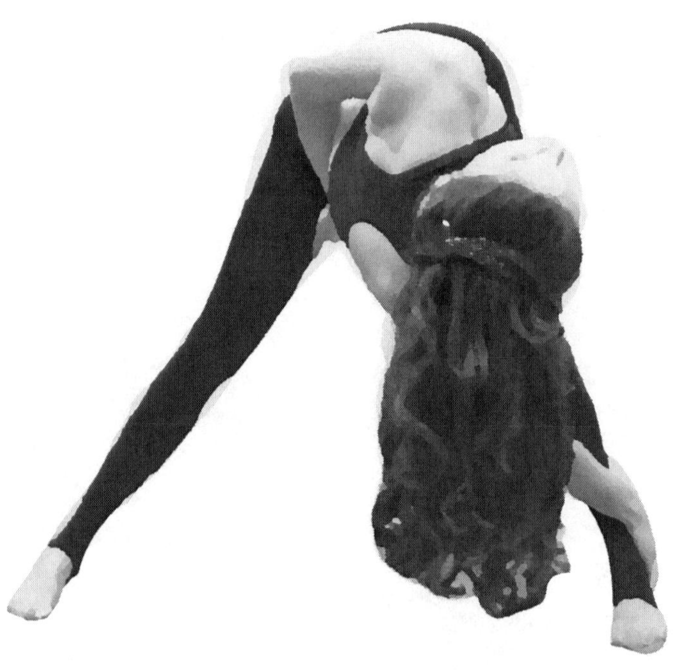

This can be anyway.
Is *this*
Flamboyant, fabulous fun?
Is *this*
Terrifying tedious tit for tat?
Is *this*

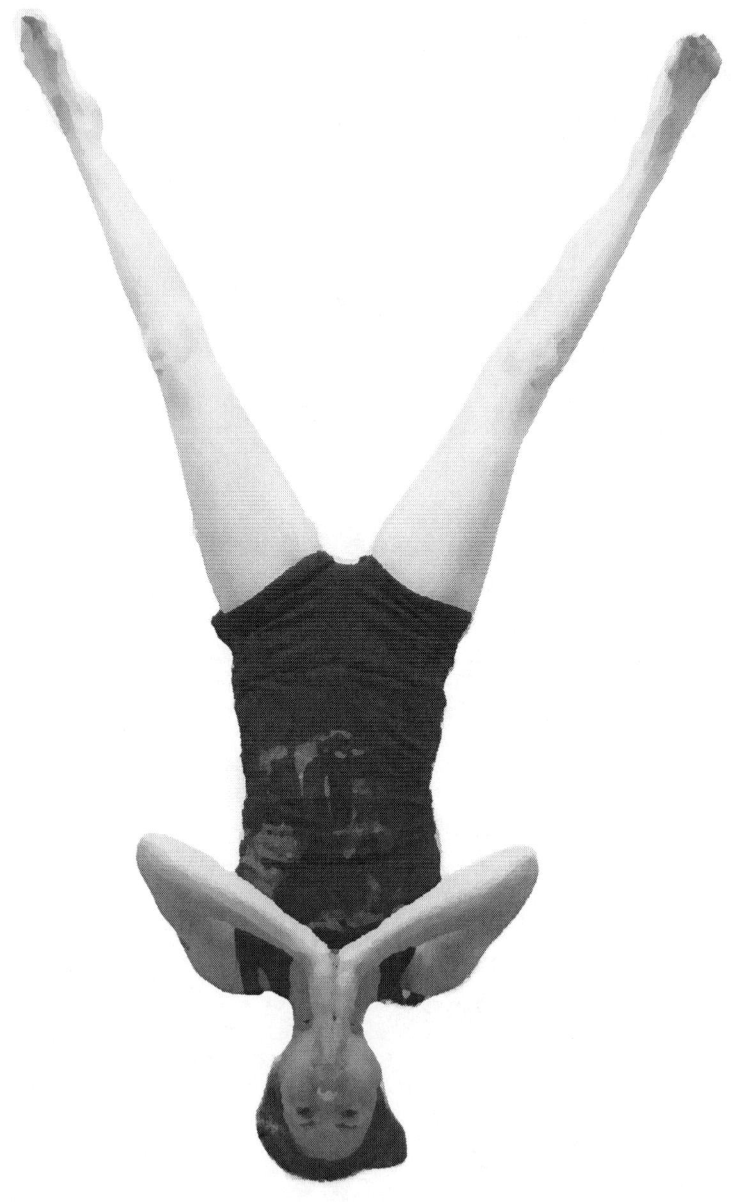

Yeah -yeah - the heart - play *that* guitar (st)ring

ok yeah i life/t my heart skywards which can accompany a feeling of rela(xa)tion in the shoulders*.

* i kno(i)w my words/ w(r)iting is genius my eyes/fingers (see) just go where they go with no direction, no plan and no agenda - legend

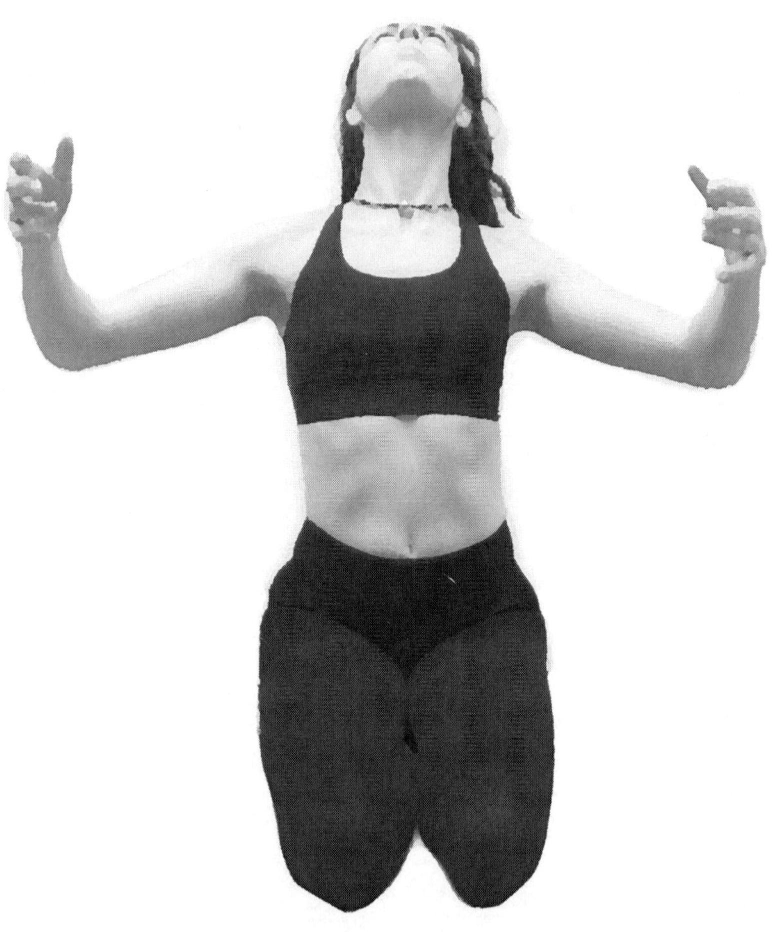

Get This

Asana, Pranayama and meditation are all here now.
Nothing is needed,

This word can be the most important word. *This* is not a direction. *This* is not a should word. There is no excuse for "beginners".

(It is possible *that this* experience is what *this* is about? Oh well - is there space in *that*? possibly a sense of duality?)

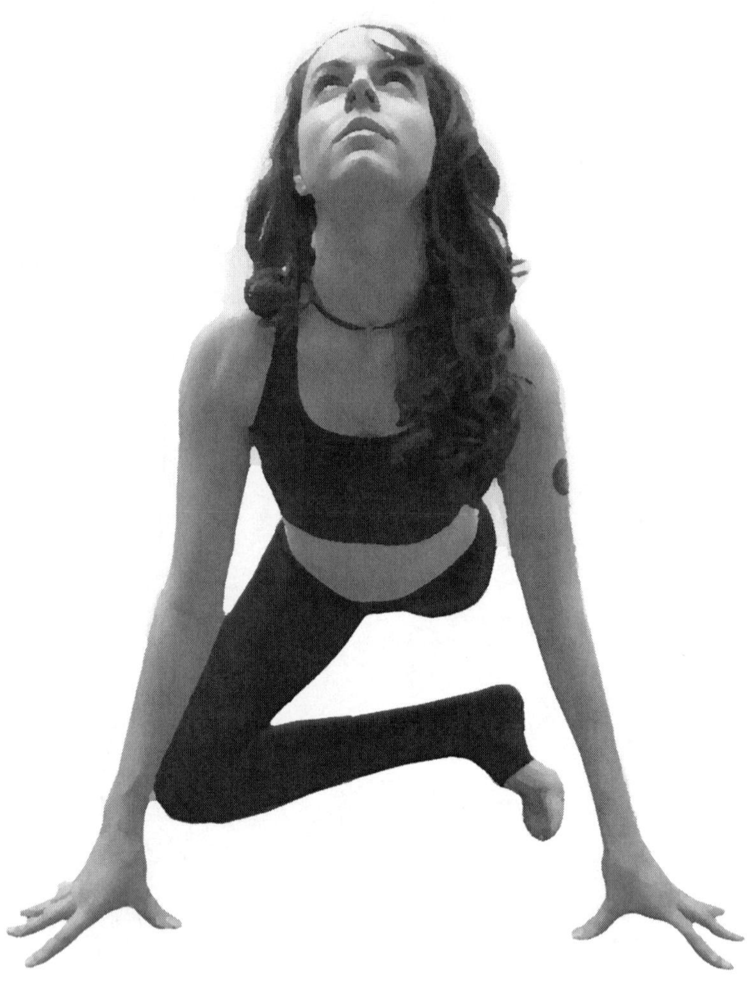

Get oneness and know everyone in *this* class knows it all!
Get *that* and there is no teacher.
Play with *that* - any face can front the CYoga class.
Get *that* - *this* is the only CYoga Qualification one requires.

No wonder CYoga classes are popular.
Everyone turns up.

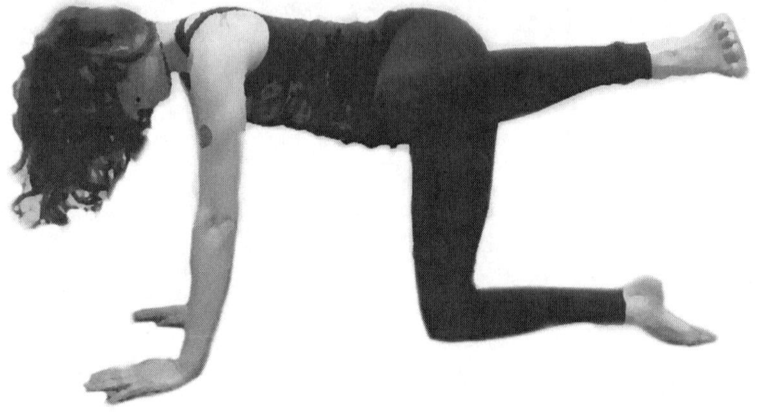

There is no separation.
Is *that* the experience now?
The Buddha position is not a requisite, unless one is in it now, for getting *that*.
This is not an advanced place to be.
There can be any sense now.
Is there a preferred sense now?
Oh well *that*'s just a sense.
Trying to compassionately accept the way it is is just a sense and one I would not seek.
Is *this that* bad *that* one wants to try to accept it and accept it with compassion? Or is (it) all one?
Now is - as it is.
Understand nothingness and free of trying.
It is NOW *that* the penny drops - not another.
It is not about accepting the way it is.
I am (in) my yoga position now.
That is it.

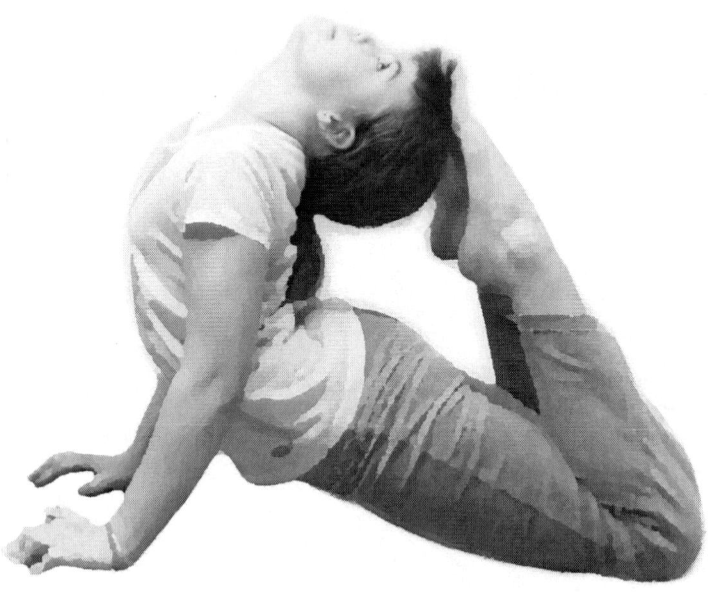

See!
Why? Oh Gee!
A.

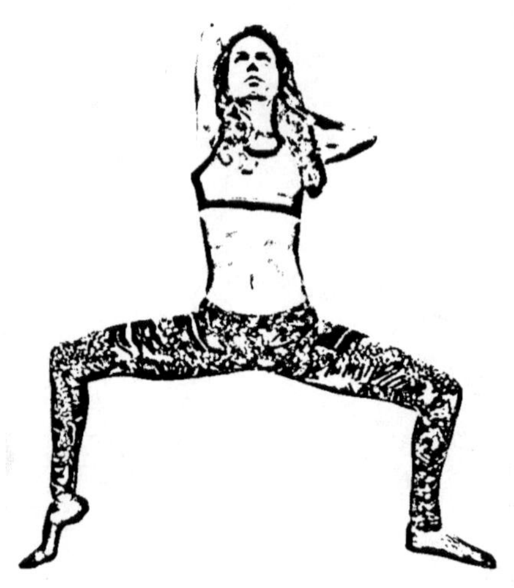

The eternal Star

See the sky.
See a star.
Do you want it?
I'll sell it.
Thanks for the payment.
Now you own *that* star.
That star is always yours.
Now you own *this* book.
This book is always yours.
Even if you don't buy it - it is yours!
This understanding is always.
This understanding is I.
There is no other.
Sky yoga.
See(a) yoga.

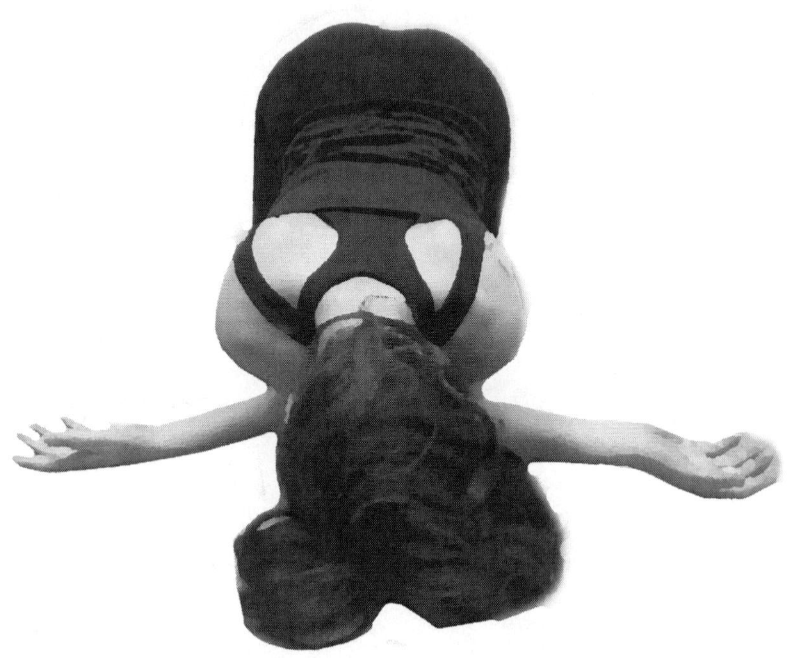

Get *that*
The understanding of *this*
Answers any questions
Dissolves any dilemmas
This space is all.

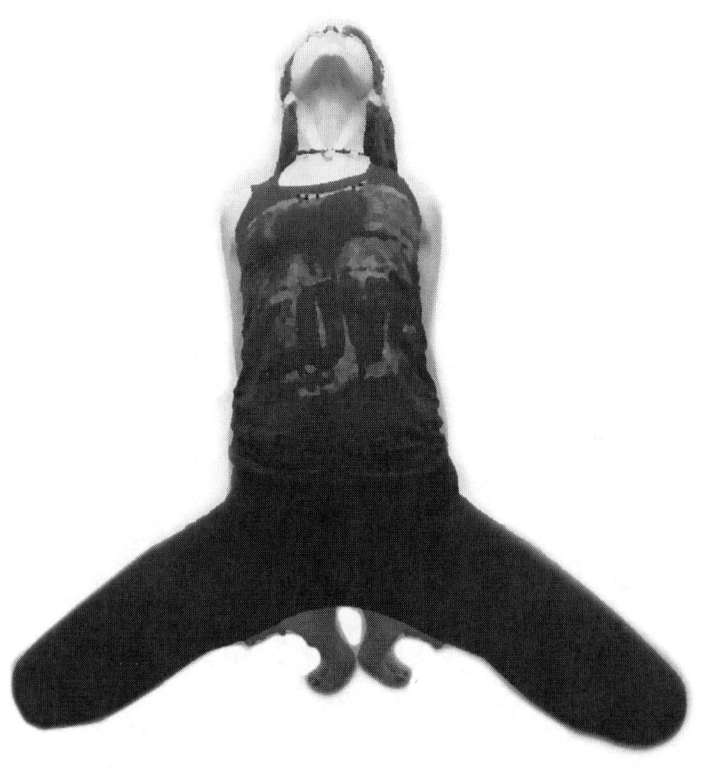

Sense the headstand

With forearms and the tip (footnote 3) of the head on the ground
Fingers spread
Pushing the forearms firmly the weight shifts from the head

Legs can be grounded or in the air.

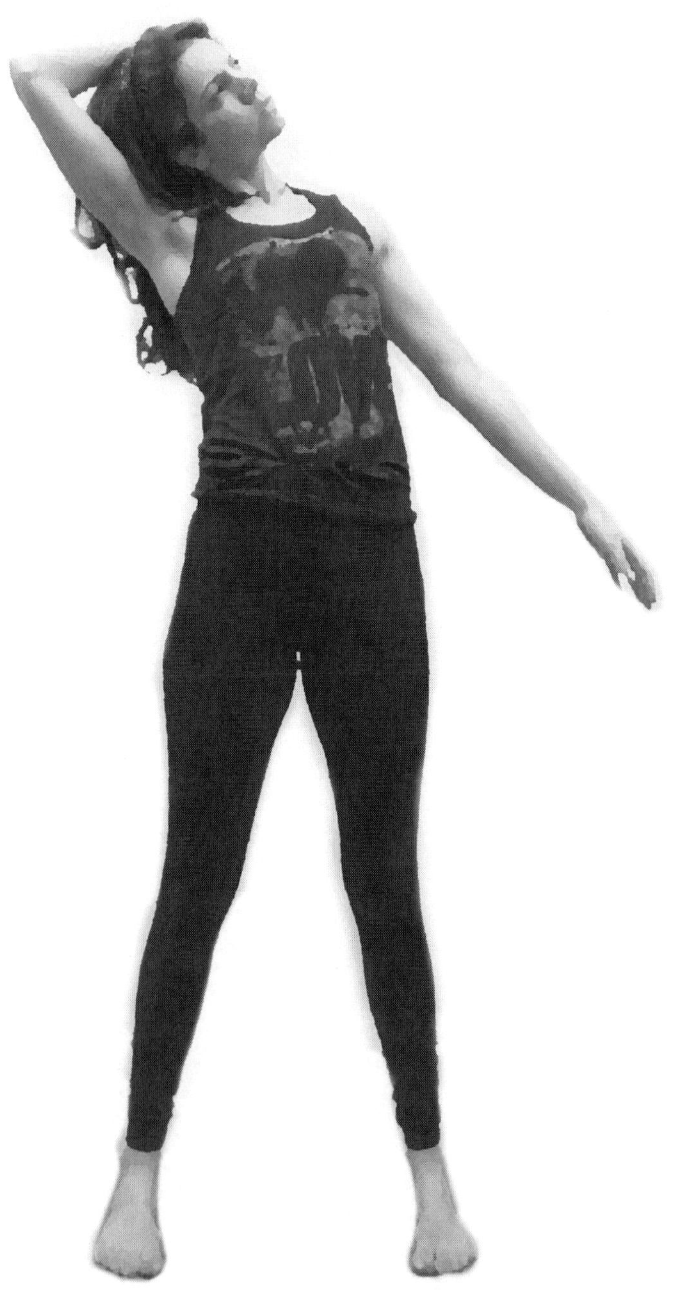

The tree of knowledge

One tree
Fruition of branches
Leaves aplenty
A branch is the tree
A leaf is the tree
A leaf is the source
A branch is the source
A leaf is the branch!
See *that*.
One shares what one knows.
One Knows.
One (is) *this*

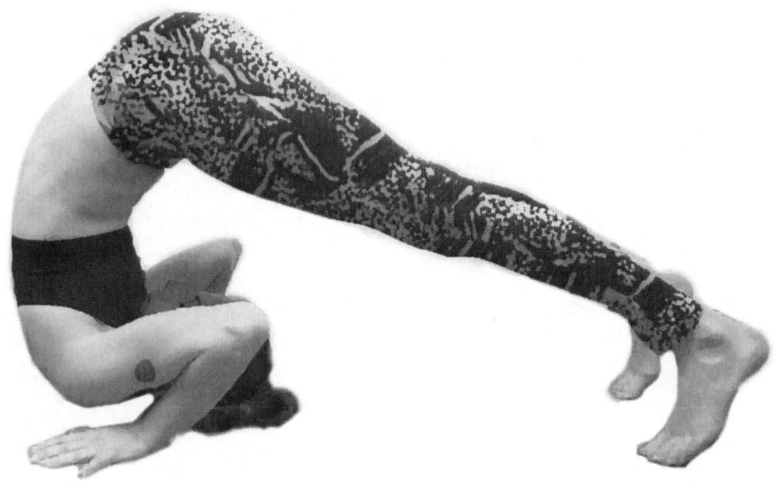

Death

Can you miss yourself?
This is the only sense.
If only?! (koan)

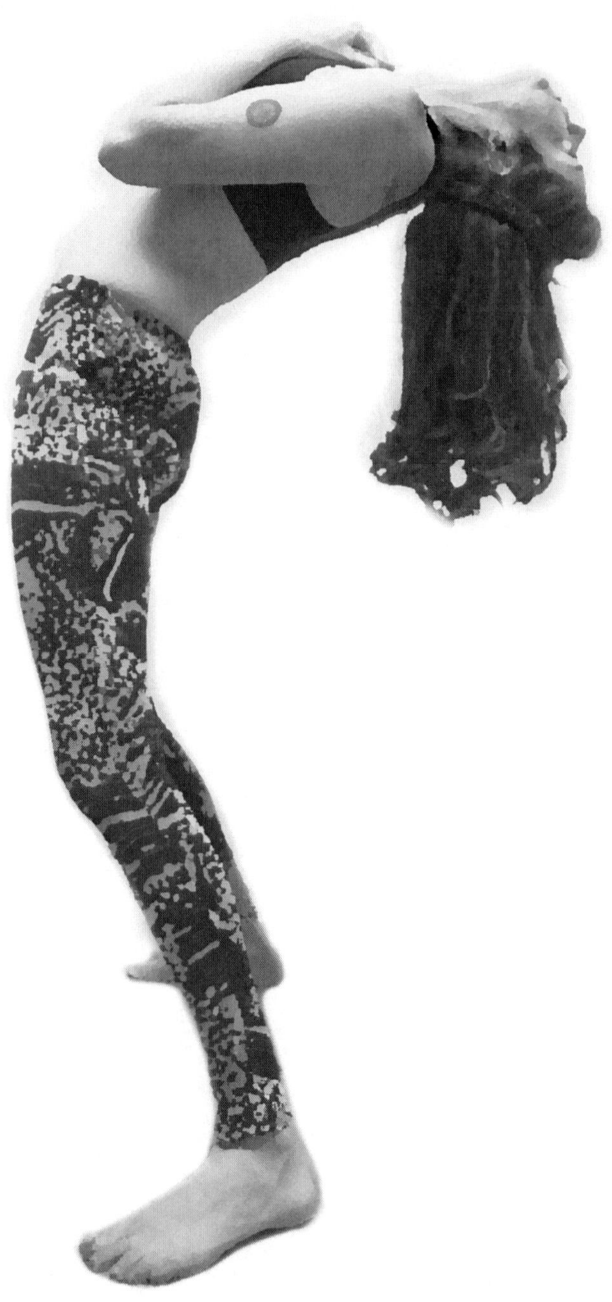

Is *that this* experience?
If not don't worry about it.
Oh the beauty of telling myself *this*.
This experience is not important.
This is one's only reference
This is one's only existence.
See *that*.
See/ be the space of *that*.

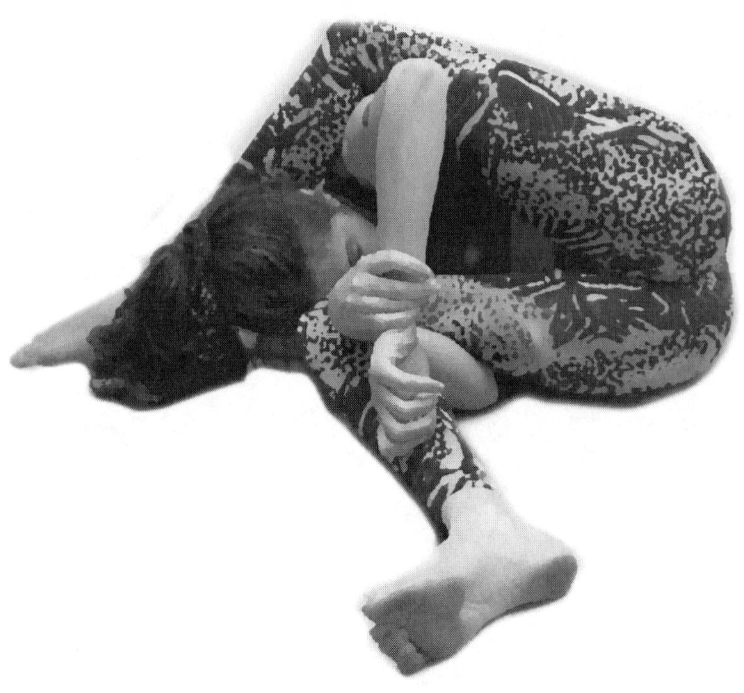

A Play on the genius of CYoga

CYoga
See Yoga
Sea Yoga
Si Yoga

Phonetically:
Ki Yoga
Key Yoga

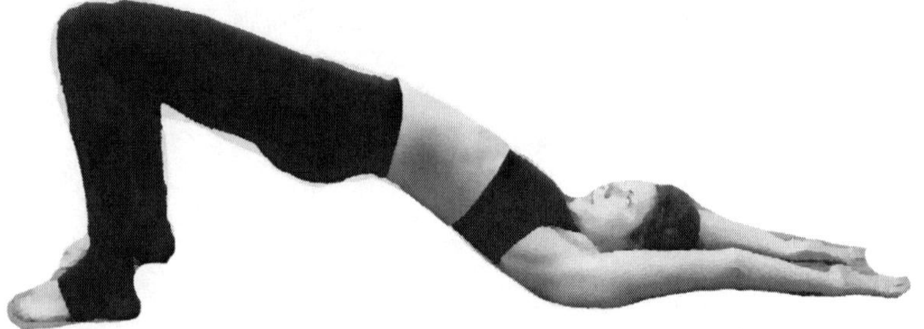

Starting Yoga

If keen to get into yoga!
I suggest loving *this* beginning.

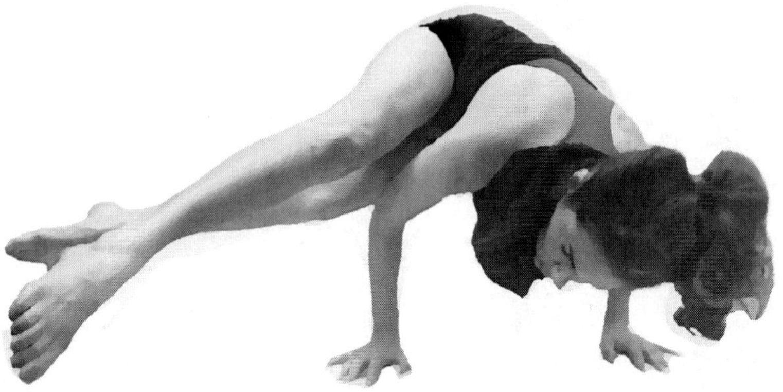

No trying

Try for what?
Anyway *this* is it
This is the point.
Anyway the benefits of no trying are relaxation and presence.
The achievements are accomplished with no try harding.

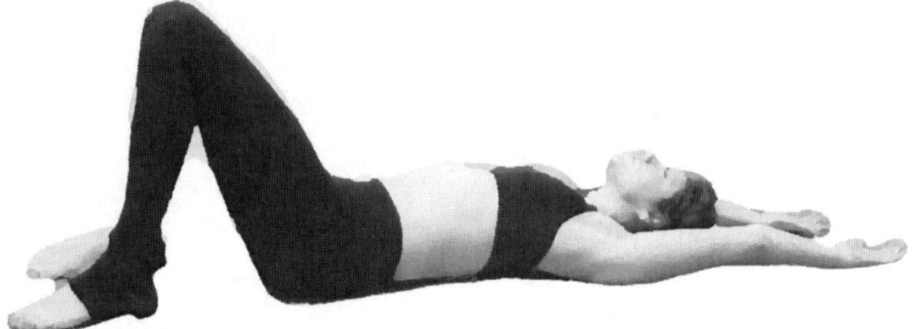

This is meditation
Why does one meditate?!
If at all.
Realise *that*.
That is meditation.
That is all.
Yes now.
The breath can be the only or the predominant attention.
This word can be the centre or the mantra.
Yes *this* is it.
Do I meditate every Morning?
Is it morning now?
It could be.
It must be if I create morning now.
Am I playing with Maya in *this* meditation?

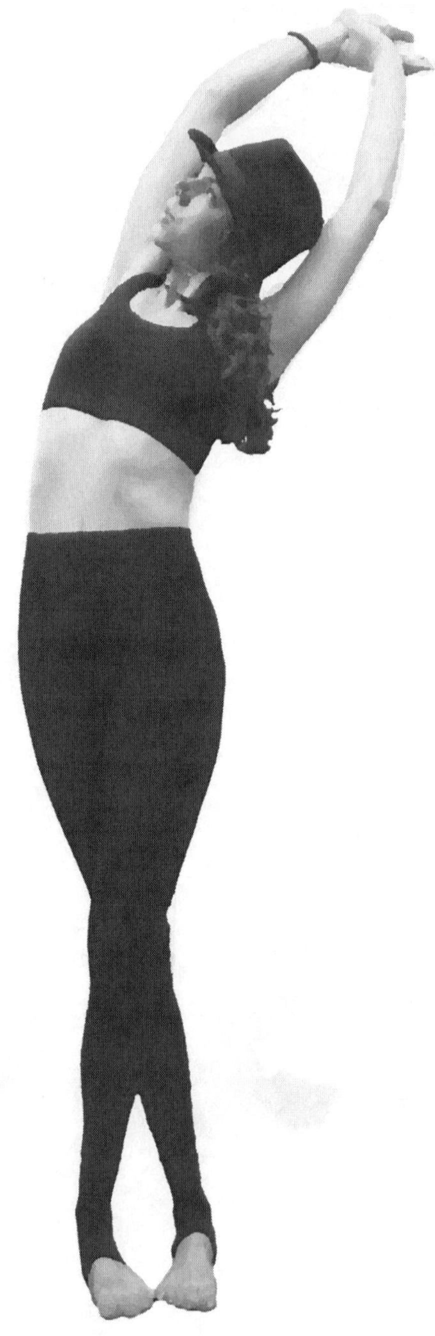

Speaking or written meditation can be "mistaken (footnote 4)" for mediation or medication. Is *that* just my experience?!

I do not meditate!

Meditation is *this*. If one is sitting quietly now reading *this that* is it.

If one is singing *this that* is it.

Understanding oneness,
undressing senses,
undressing thoughts.
One knows what one knows everyone knows.
One knows what one does everyone can do.
See the joke(footnote 5) in differing opinions.
See the joke (footnote 6) in differing abilities.
Splits anyone?

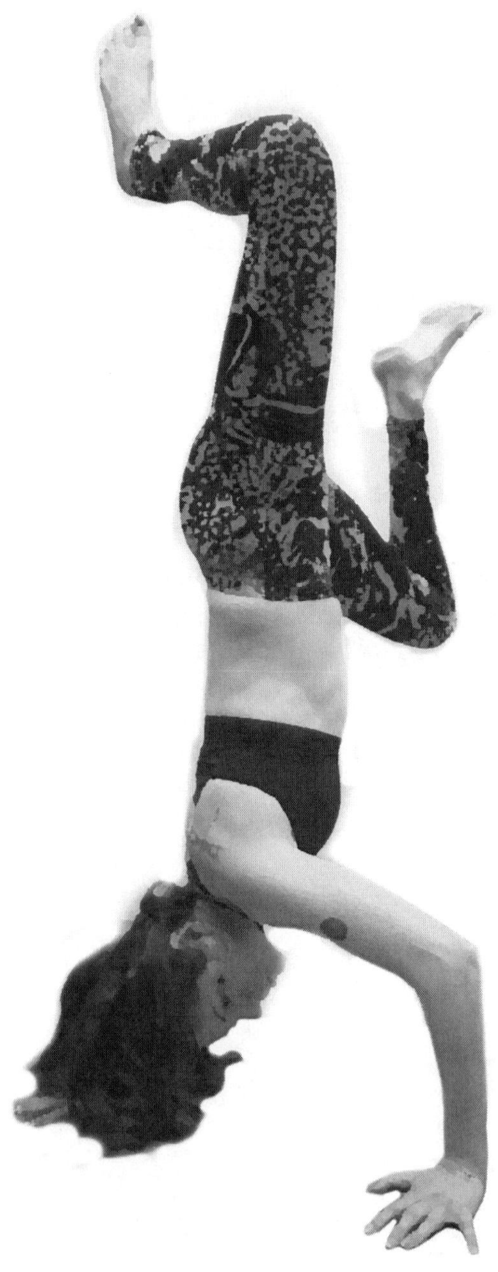

Do not worry about what the body does.
The "thought system" does not need to understand.

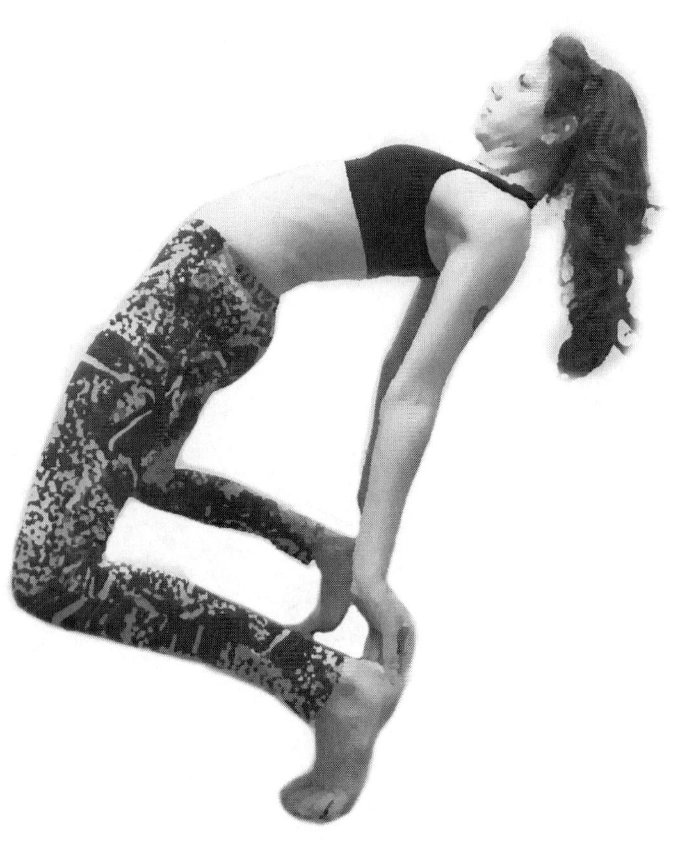

This is the essence of CYoga
This is always the art
It is not learn some notes to make a symphony *that* is one's own.
This symphony is always one's own.
Get It?!
Of course - you are me!

I sing without learning the notes - A, B, C.
I read without learning the letters - A, B, C.
There is no learning.

How easy is *this*?!
This symphony is (in) harmony.

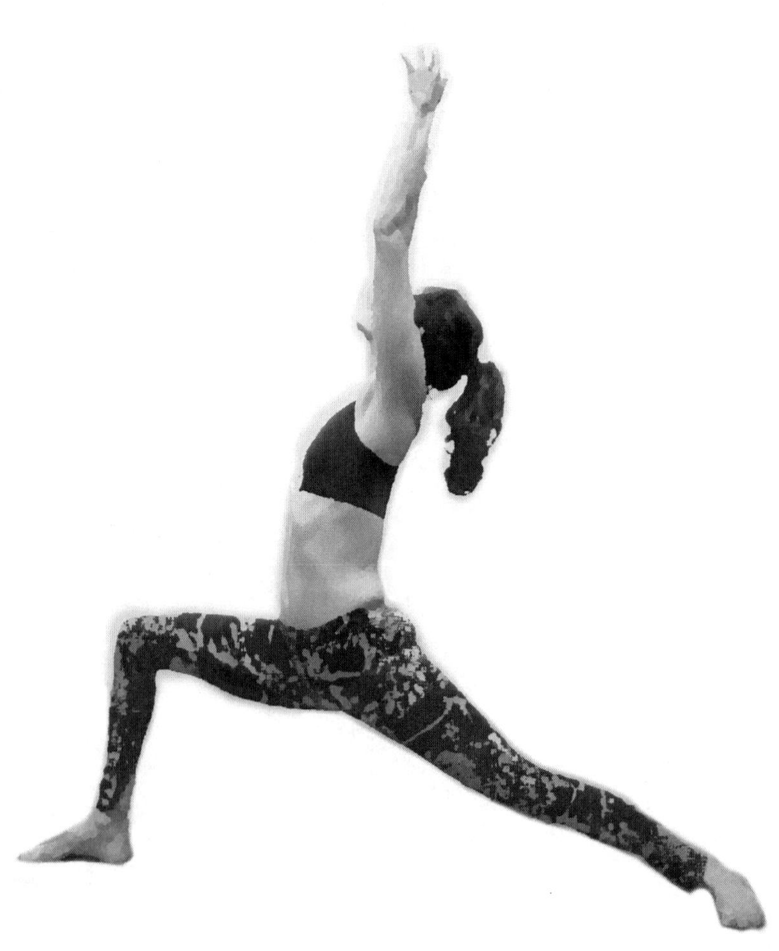

CYoga an be hath yoga
Astanga yoga
Vinyasa yoga
Fluid yoga
Meditation
Pranayama
Yin Yoga
Yang yoga
Jazz
Contemporary dance
Capoiera
Tai chi
Jujitsu
Juu jitsu (don't ask!)
Belly dancing
African dance
Hip hop!
ballet
any more (your/my choice)
How can *this* be?!
All a body in a position
Understand oneself
All is possible.

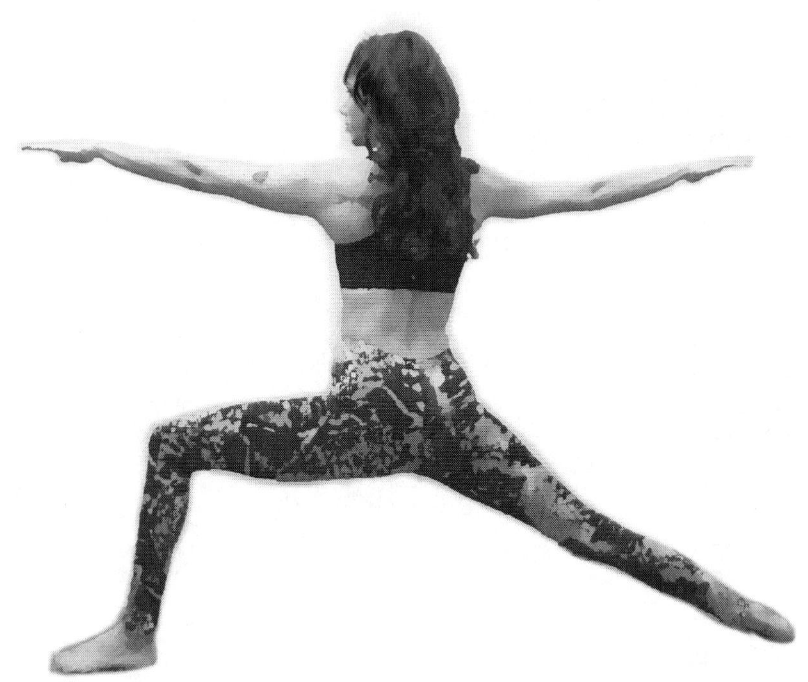

Be all the chart.
That is a yogic chart.
That can be a yogic art.
Method acting anyone?
That is it.

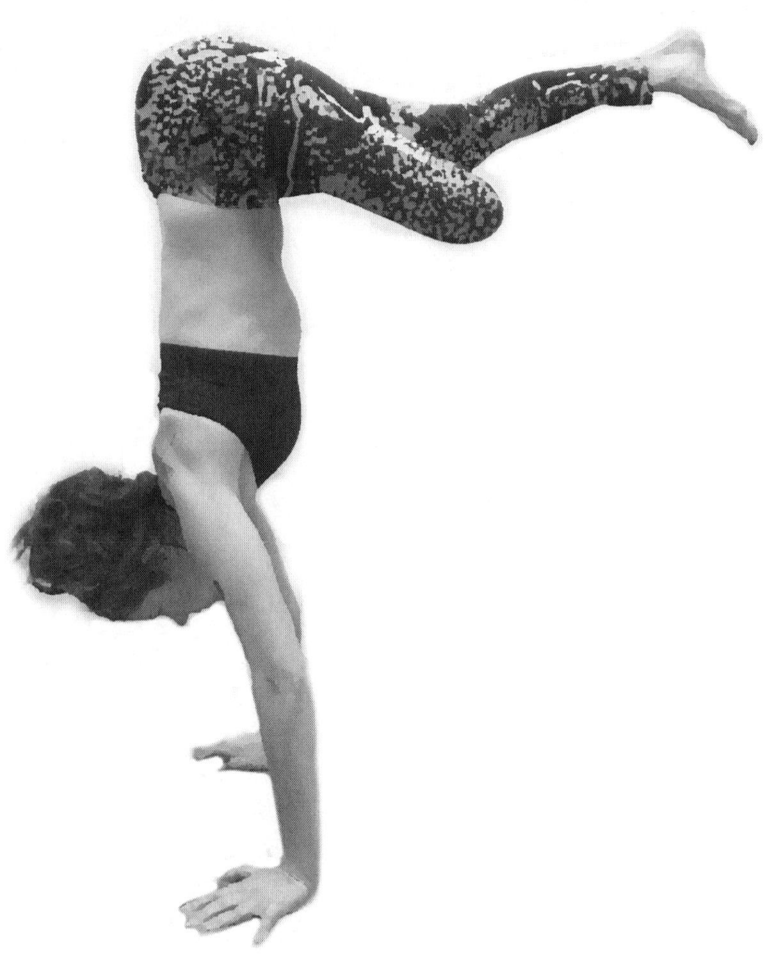

It

You're it!
I dare you to catch me.
Caught up yet?!

(cheat - *This* Is It Game)

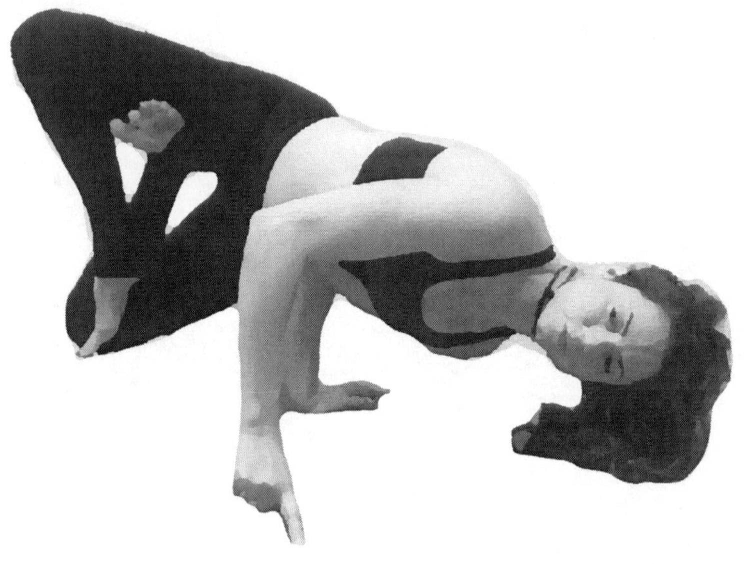

Yoga is all
Get *that*.
You can be every characteristic.
You can be every face.
This word can be you.
This word is me.

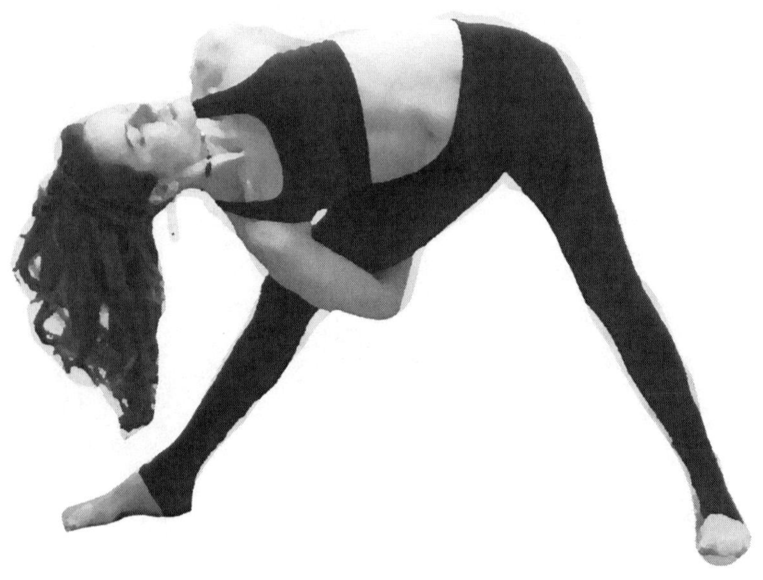

Feelings/ senses can be seductive/ all encompassing

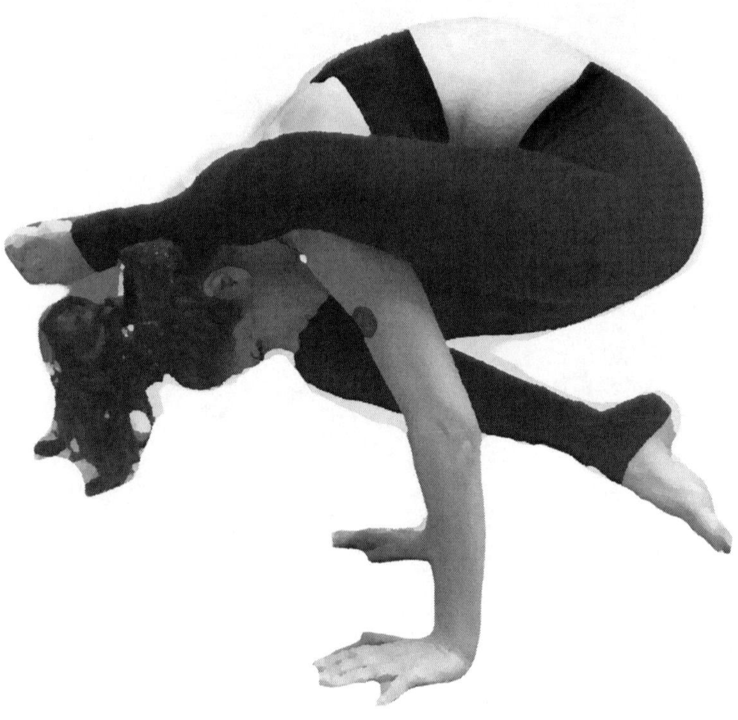

This is a yoga manual.
Who wants *that*?
This is the best how to get into a position book/word.
The position is *this*.
How easy is *that*?
Get it?!

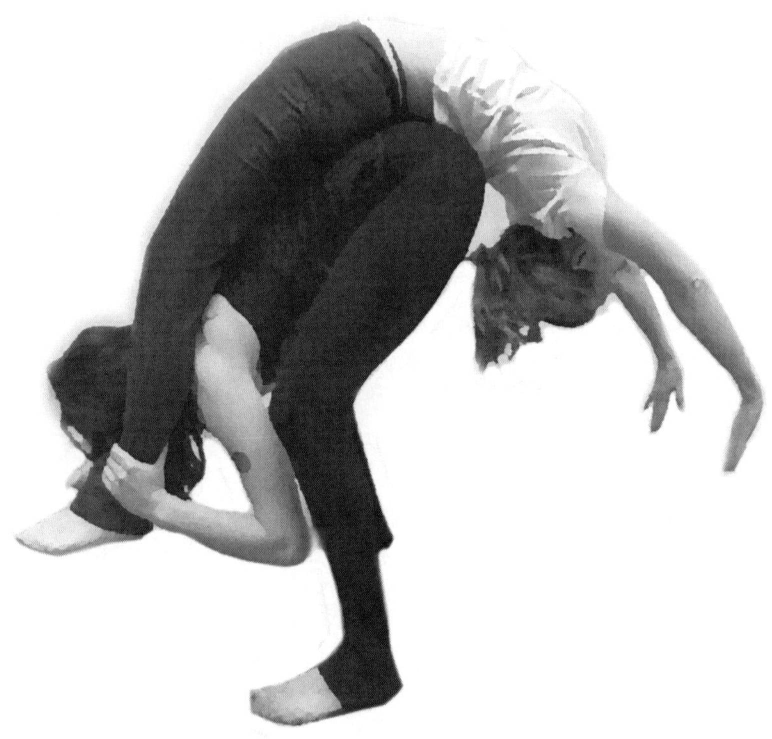

With *this* CYoga class
Is *that* the culmination of CYoga?!
What an orgasm. *This* is as good as it gets

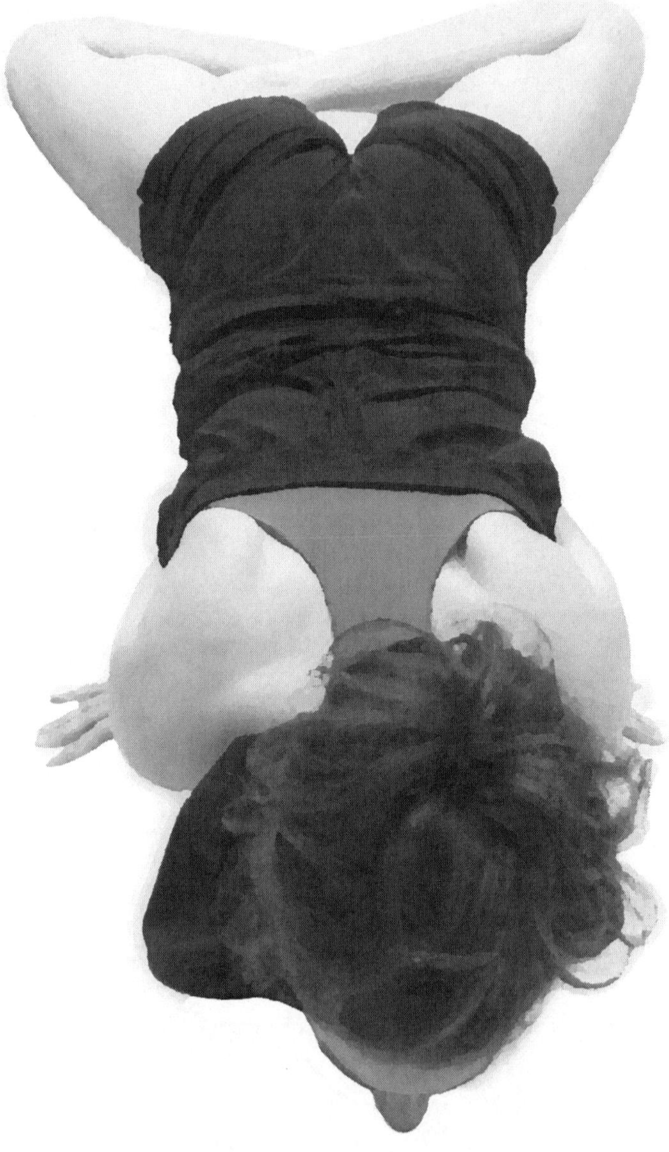

CYoga is as it is.
It is not necessary to do something to (a) achieve CYoga
The idea of "oh with practice I get it" can present.
The easiest option is one has (it) all now!
It is not necessary to prove a feat is attainable by you/ I.
You/ I am is a one armed handstand now.
How it looks is not important.
Regardless of what presents know you are Champion of any CYoga position.

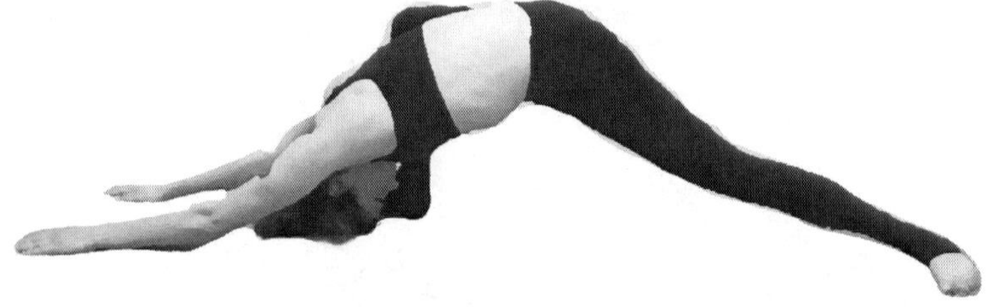

CYoga

Speaking Sanskrit with no prior training is possible.
Being the no 1 martial artist with no experience is possible.

Get it - one is/has all - no sucking is necessary for victory in any/all fields.
Be Victor (Hoo…go!)

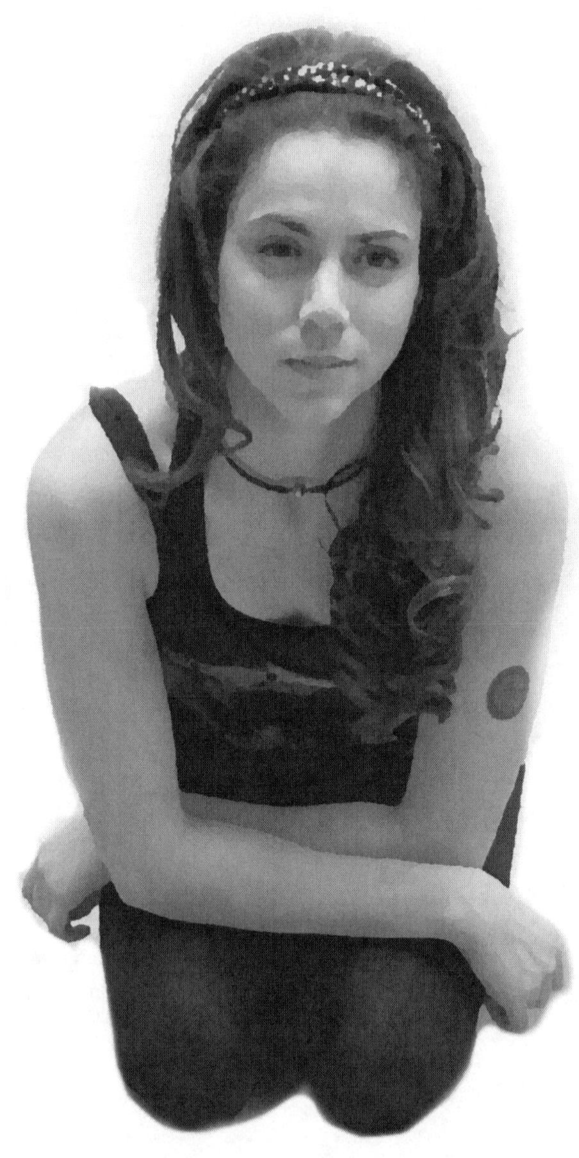

There can be a sense of achievement.
There can be a sense *that this* is a challenge.
There can be a sense of evolvement.
There can be (a) sense *That This* Is It.
There can be (A) sense of how sense is created Now.

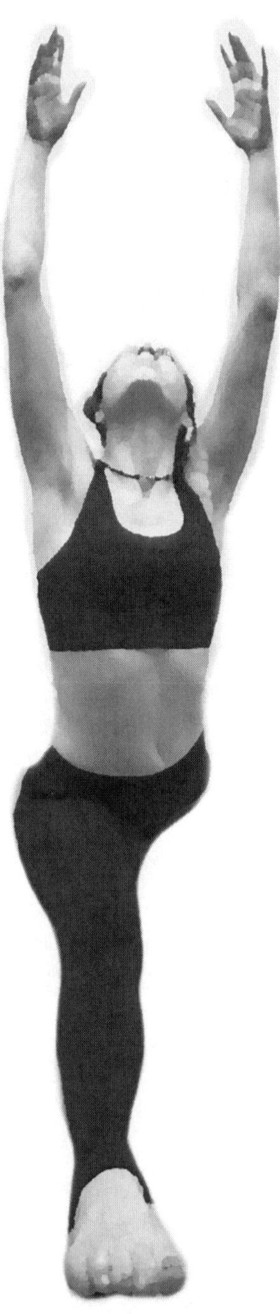

There is no random m(e) movement.

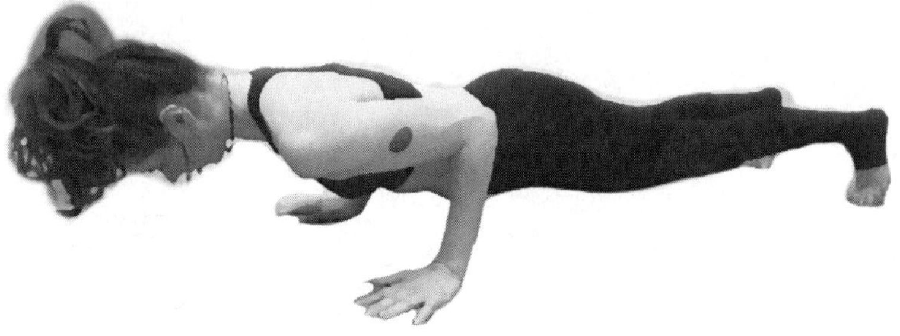

Is Yoga Indian?!
Are you Indian?
Am I Indian?
Is *this* Indian?
Perhaps Yoga is Brazilian. (I love capoiera or just I!)
Perhaps Yoga is Hollywood.

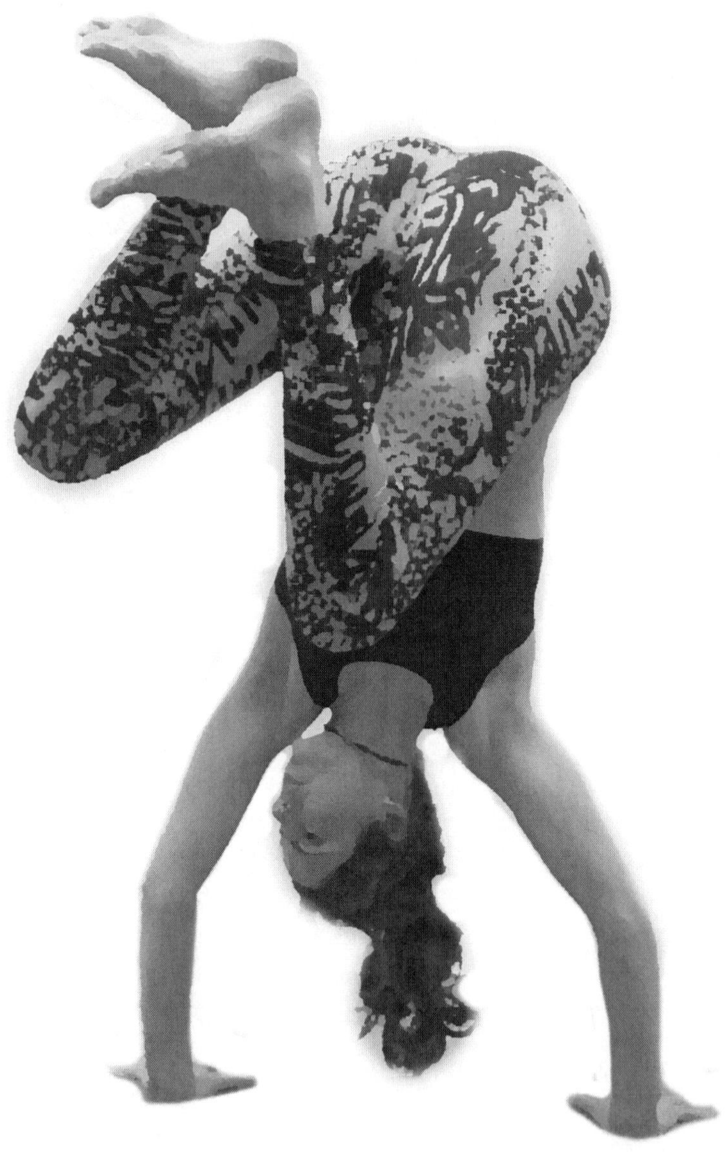

What is (a) yoga (teacher)?
How should I qualify myself?!
Can one teach one what is always known?
One can pretend *that* there is an "other one".
Let's call the other one "student".
So the other one "student" can learn yoga from the one.
How wonderful!
By creating the other one the one shows the other one *that* the other one is always a student of the one!
Is the other one a step away from being Boss?!
Can the other one be yoga?!
Being a student is the subject not fully known?
Is the other one not being one?!
Be yoga.
See yoga.
If one is a teacher is there something t(w)o teach?
The CYoga class is an open class.
Be a know all - even if one does not know.
There is no other.
There is no teacher.
There is no student.
There is no subject.
There is no drama.
Yeah I know all *this*.

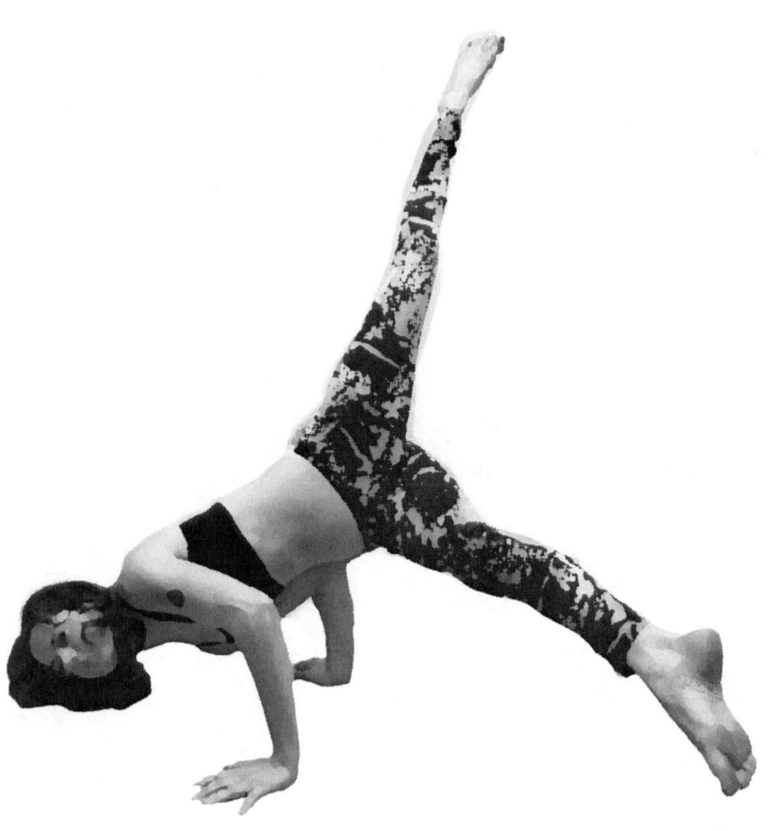

See if there is a witness to *this*.
See if there is a witness to *this* thought.
See if there is a witness to any feelings such as clothing contact, temperature, the sense of ground.
Is there only one?
Is there a sense of more than one?
What is one?
There is only I.
This is all.

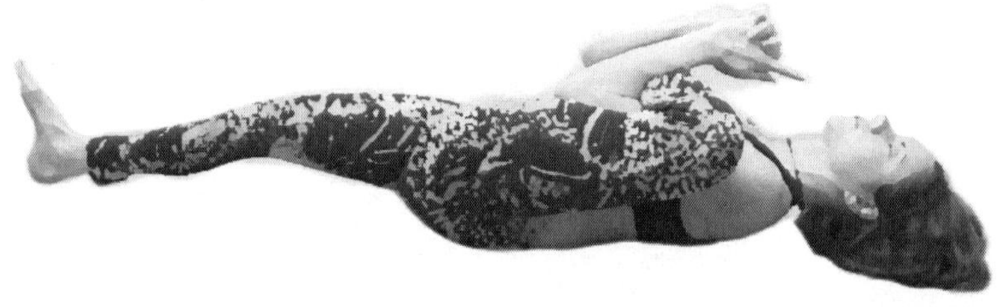

There are no coincidences!
It may appear *this* is one. (Get *that* - double entendre!)

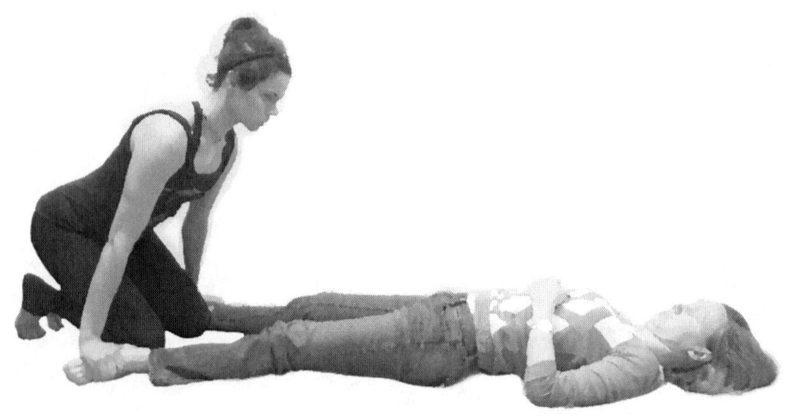

This is not "forgetting any story".
There is no story.
This is not letting go of any story.
There is no story.
This can be being Here Now and dropping any labels such as "I am *This*" (woman/man/ African/ English/lawyer/ postman/ dancer/ strong/ tall etc.) or I am *That*.
There are no labels.
What is the sense now?
This is the only sense.
There is nothing *that* requires doing Now.
Here is all.
There can be understanding *that* Now is all.
There can be understanding *that* Now - the creation of Sense - is Here.
With *This* one can have/be anything and everything.

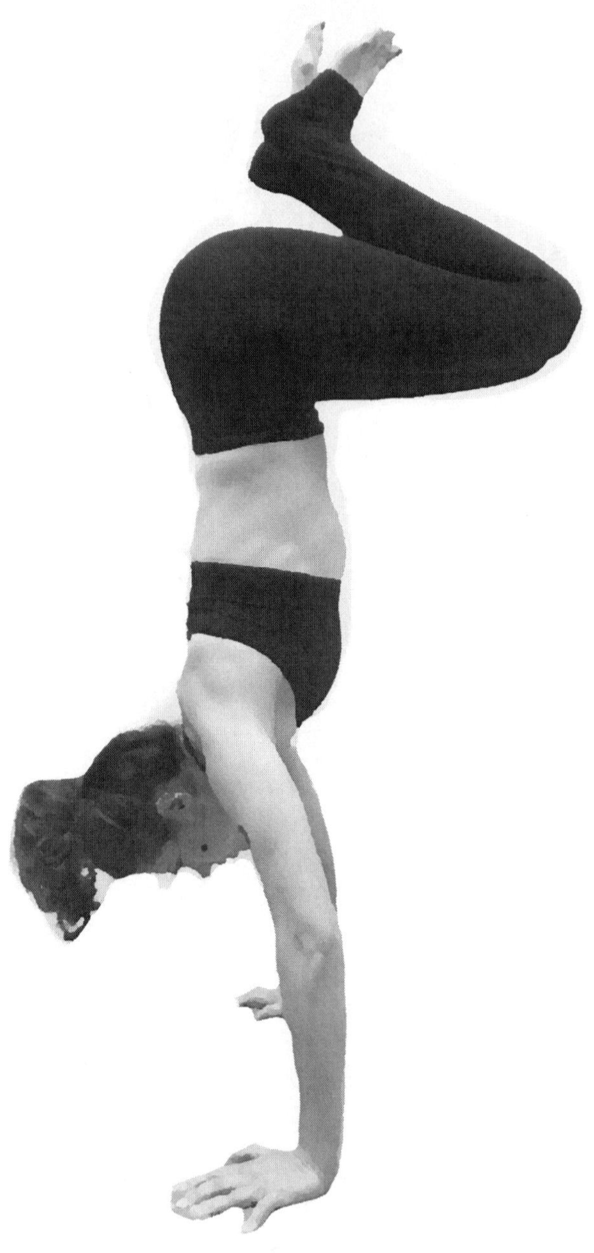

Describing *this* as meditative or Taoist is really too much! It is just *this*.

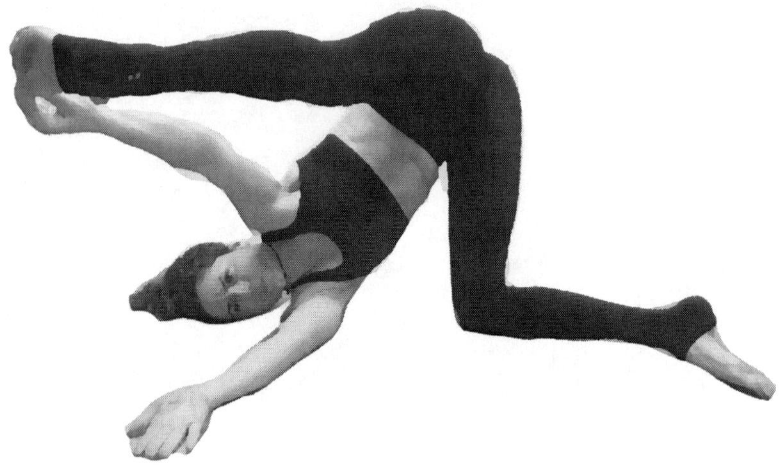

Yippeeeee.

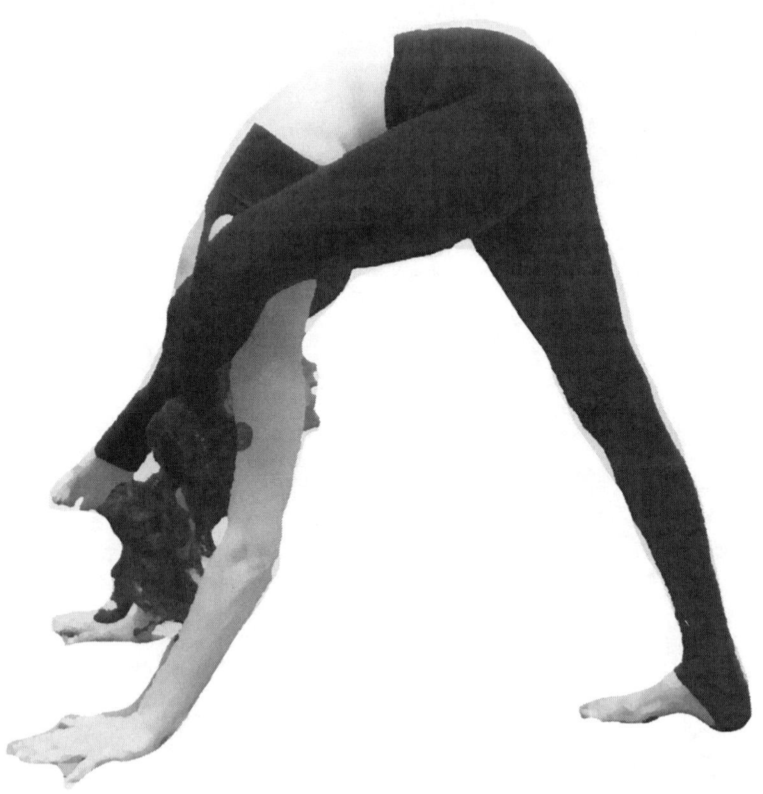

Naked of roles and image.
Naked of all
 - shape shifting can present.
Correction - there is only *this* shape.

What shape is *this*?!

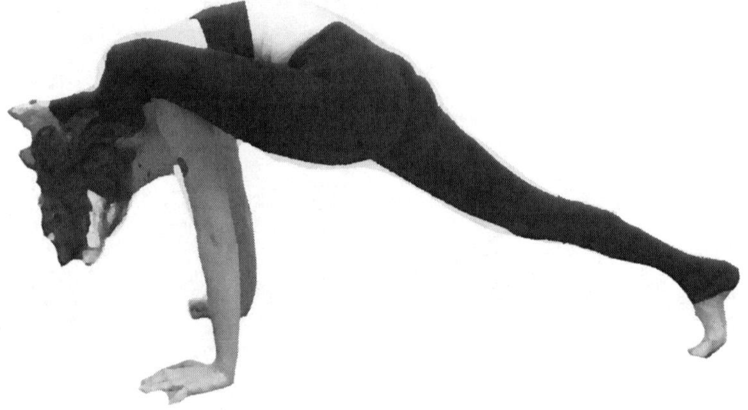

The C stands for cheeky - cheeky yoga - gotta love it!

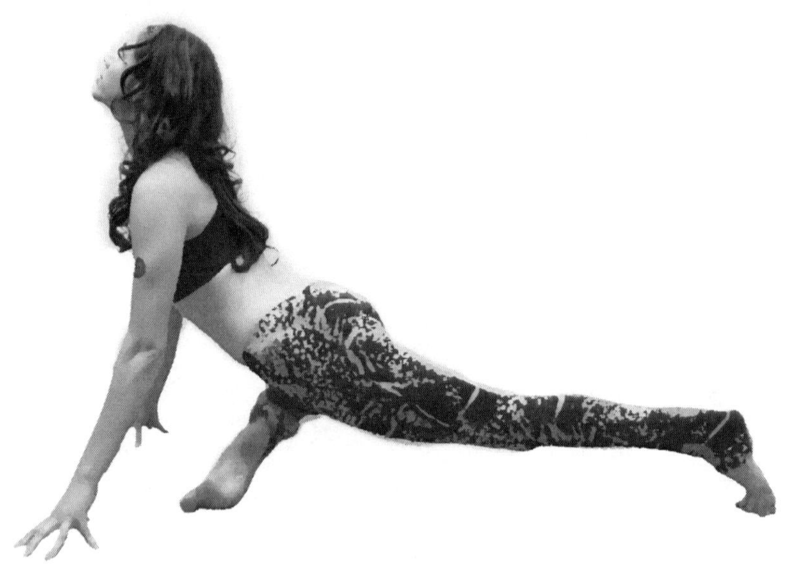

I can present yoga.
This is It?
Easy.

How on Earth can I teach it (footnote 7)?!
Perhaps in heaven.

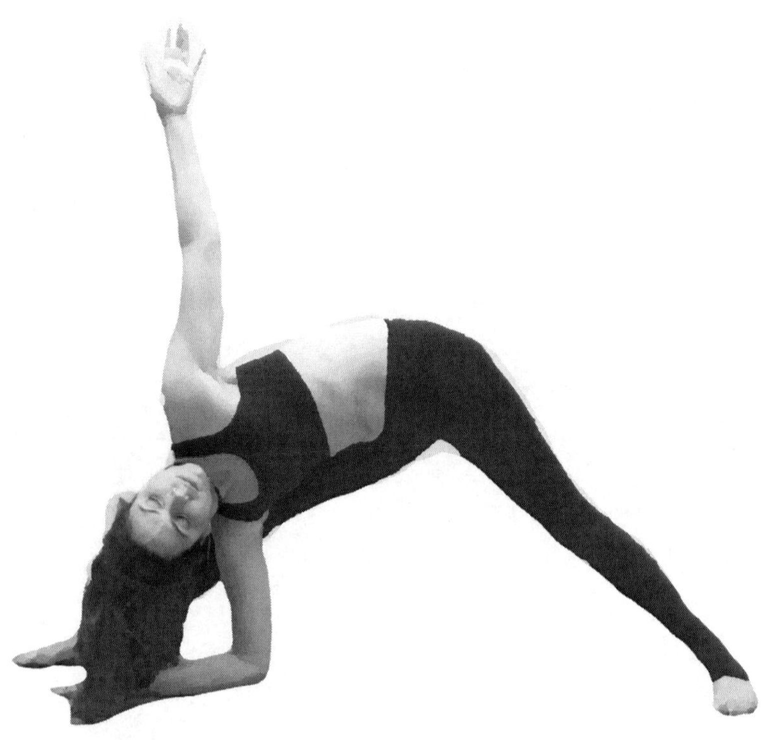

With the understanding of *this* one gets *that* all days are here now and one creates it *this* way.

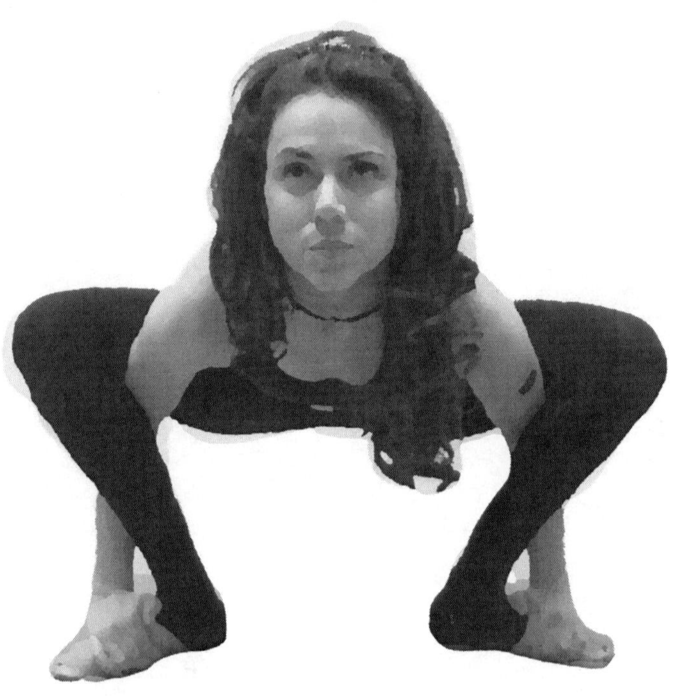

One sees/is the illusion of being present and knowledge *that* one has everything now - whatever *that* is = is Maya.

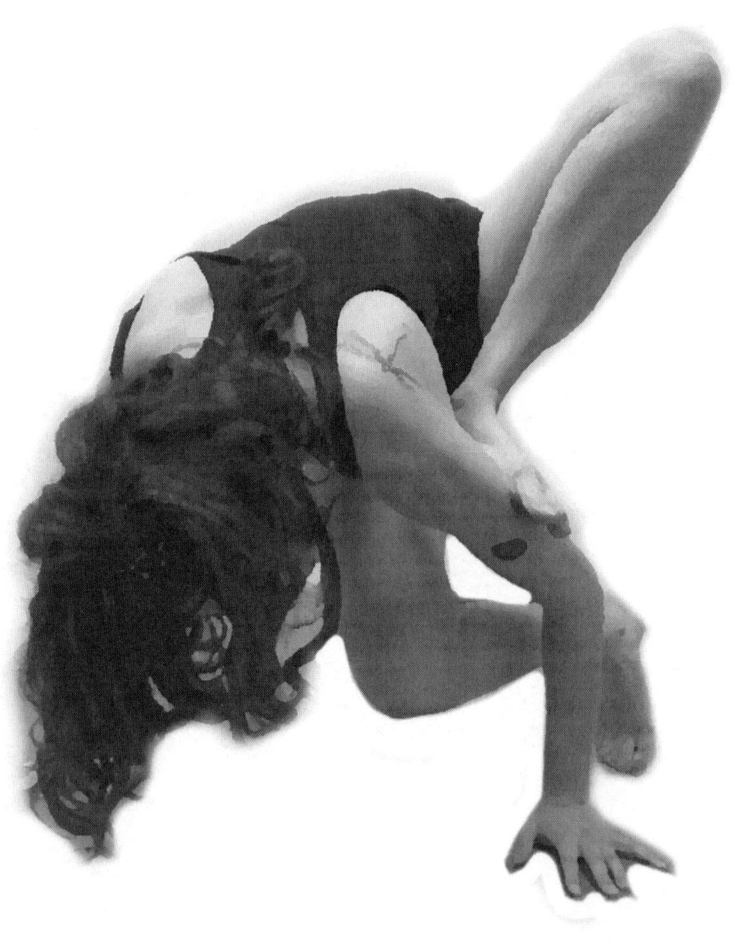

This is what Katie gets up to next!

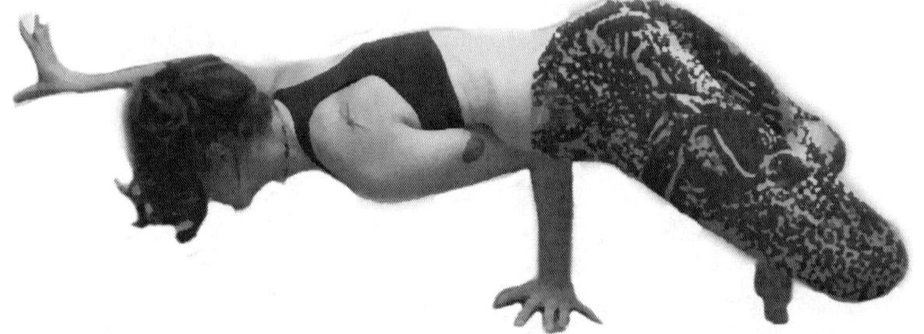

How long have I been yoga?

The feeling is forever.

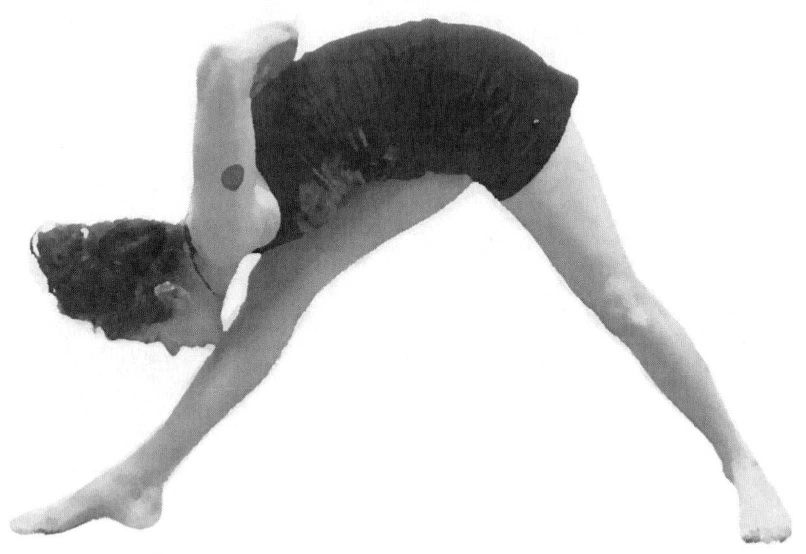

I am brilliant at detailing *this* position/ yoga asana's inner/ external anatomical/ physiological structure and senses/I; and tipping.

Get *that*.
So are you.
The owning of *this* experience can be everything.
I share *that this* experience is created by you/ I and *this* is you/ I.
What position am I in now?
This is enough.
Truly yours.

This is It II (aye aye).

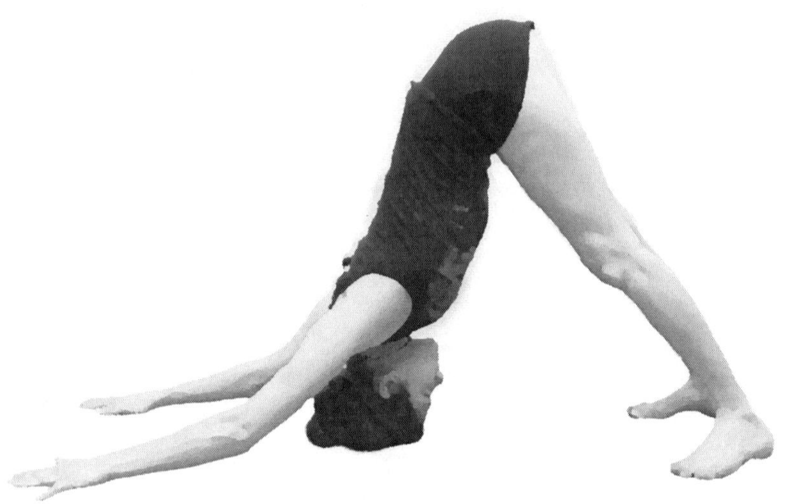

Tip

Understand Maya.
Be.
This is the territory to be any shape.

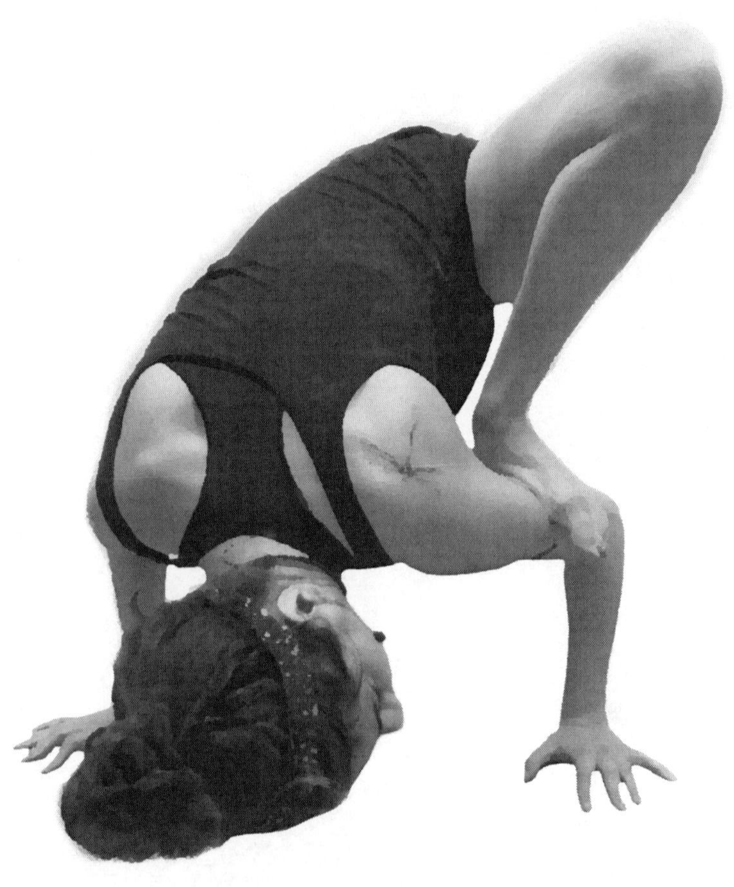

Who Wrote *This* It II - Enlightenment With CYoga?

You-I!

Are you Catherine Foroughi?!

"I am *This*."

"You/ I are/am *This*"

CYoga Creator; Yoga Therapist, Lawyer; Choreographer; CYoga Body Architect; Author; Artist.

This is I.

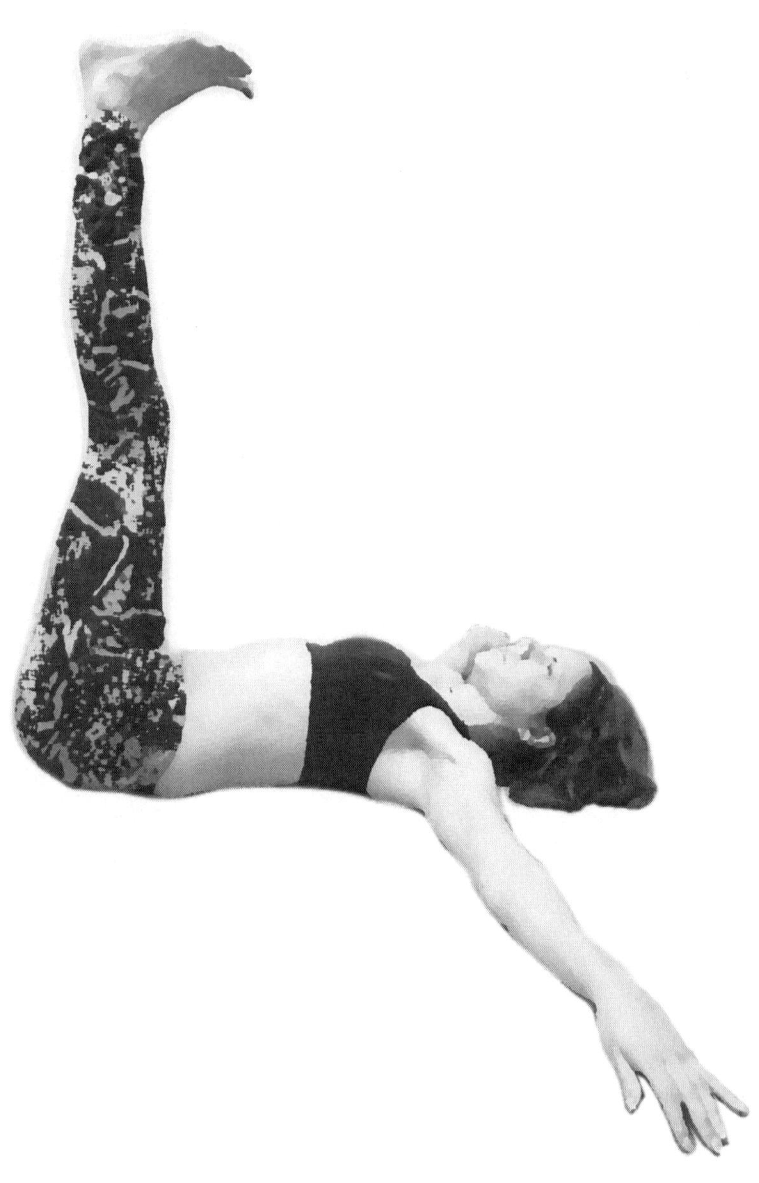

About CYoga

CYoga can be seen as yoga, a dance and/or a martial art. Simply CYoga is *This*. There are no boundaries.

The CYoga Art is integrated and interactive. One can mention the interplay of three energies and principles.
The energies are playing with *this*, working with *this* and seeing through *this*.
The three principles are:
1. the feeling of the ground
2. a sense of space
3. the utilisation of cross energy!

This CYoga class is transmission of the CYoga essence. If one understands/ is the essence of CYoga the asana/ position is always perfect.

CYoga engages in one- one's, teacher tuition, satsang/ mediation, public classes, workshops, holidays and seminars. CYoga inspires, guides and teaches "the teacher" (including yoga, dance and martial art teachers). *This* tuition is beyond discipline.

CYoga can be seen as yoga, a dance and/or a martial art. Simply CYoga is *This*. There are no boundaries.
CYoga shows the essence of yoga *that* is beyond style.
CYoga can involve; yoga asanas; breathwork (pranayama); pilates; t'ai chi; energy work (qigong); martial artistry; voice and dance work. *This* allows one all abilities. *This* is it.

For information on CYoga, tuition, seminars and workshops see: www.cyoga.co.uk and/or *This* Is It: Enlightenment With CYoga.

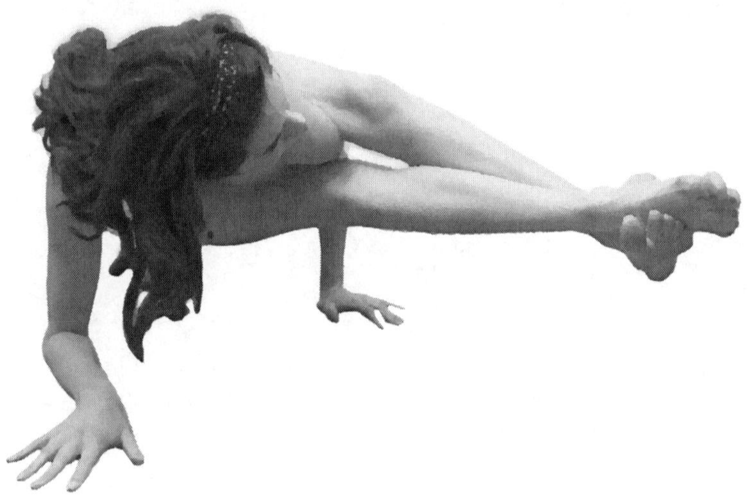

Email : See@cyoga.co.uk

That's all folks.

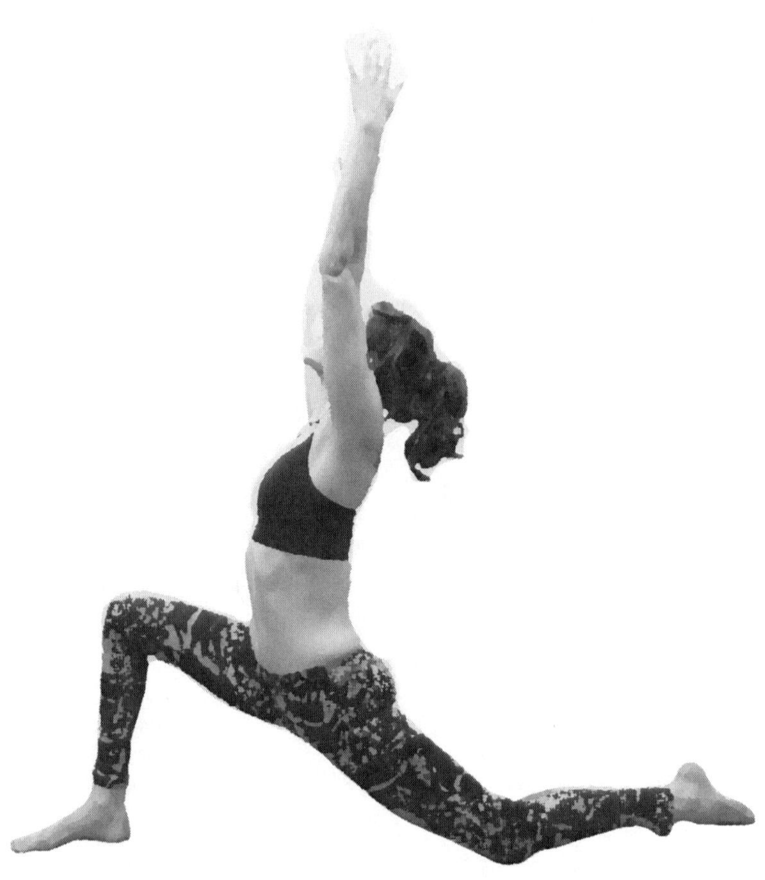

Footnotes

Footnote 1 I don't keep time. Did it ever exist? (see *This* is It Game) Do I create it now?
Footnote 2 Plank with knees on the ground is an alternative.
Footnote 3 Fontanelle and around *that* region is a good place to begin. With confidence, security and stability the position can be adjusted. Without one of these three senses it is possible.
Footnote 4 there are no mistakes?!
Footnote 5 it may not be funny
Footnote 6 it may be funny
Footnote 7 *This* Is It Game! Game Over.

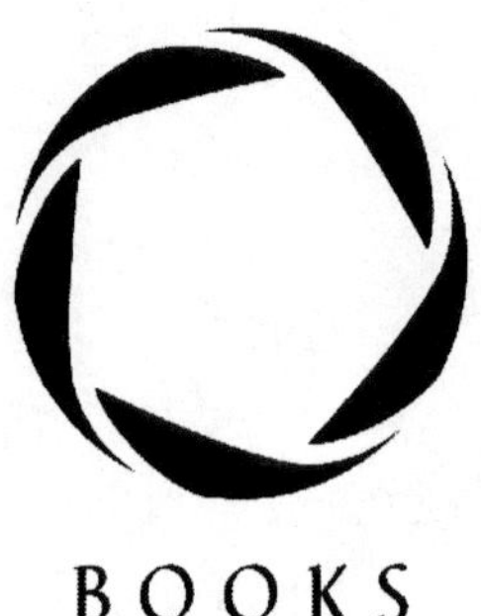

BOOKS

O is a symbol of the world, of oneness and unity. In different cultures it also means the "eye," symbolizing knowledge and insight. We aim to publish books that are accessible, constructive and that challenge accepted opinion, both that of academia and the "moral majority."

Our books are available in all good English language bookstores worldwide. If you don't see the book on the shelves ask the bookstore to order it for you, quoting the ISBN number and title. Alternatively you can order online (all major online retail sites carry our titles) or contact the distributor in the relevant country, listed on the copyright page.

See our website **www.o-books.net** for a full list of over 500 titles, growing by 100 a year.

And tune in to myspiritradio.com for our book review radio show, hosted by June-Elleni Laine, where you can listen to the authors discussing their books.

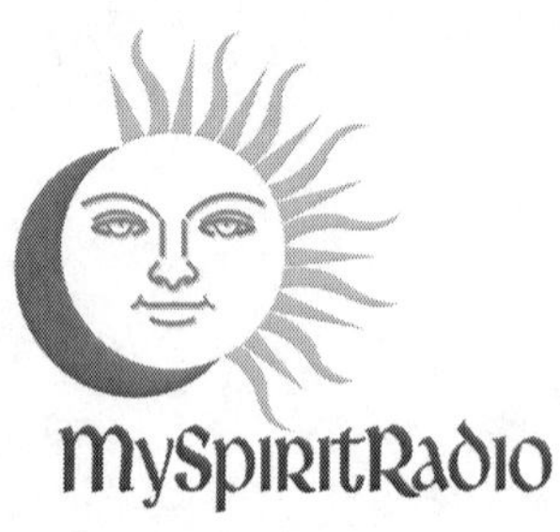